Pesticides

Communication, Environment, Science and Society Set

coordinated by
Andrea Catellani and Céline Pascual Espuny

Volume 4

Pesticides

Pluridisciplinary Dialogues in Social and Human Sciences

Edited by

Nataly Botero
Hélène Ledouble
François Allard-Huver

iSTE

WILEY

First published 2024 in Great Britain and the United States by ISTE Ltd and John Wiley & Sons, Inc.

ISTE Ltd
27-37 St George's Road
London SW19 4EU
UK

www.iste.co.uk

John Wiley & Sons, Inc.
111 River Street
Hoboken, NJ 07030
USA

www.wiley.com

Library of Congress Control Number: 2024946270

British Library Cataloguing-in-Publication Data
A CIP record for this book is available from the British Library
ISBN 978-1-78630-950-1

Contents

Author Presentation

Editors

François Allard-Huver

François Allard-Huver is an Associate Professor in strategic and digital communication at Université Catholique de l'Ouest, Angers (UCO). His work focuses on environmental and health controversies surrounding food and pesticides. He is particularly interested in the question of "affairs" in the media and the public sphere. He also works on risks, sustainable development and organizations, with a particular focus on the CSR communication and public relations strategies of various players in the public sphere (institutions, civil society, lobbies, industry). He regularly participates in symposia and conferences on the relationship between sustainable development, risks, controversy, food and communication.

A member of the management committee of the *Communication, environnement, science et société* (CESS) study and research group of the *Société française des sciences de l'information et de la communication*[1], he is also the scientific director of the *Académie des controverses et de la communication sensible* (ACCS)[2].

Nataly Botero

Nataly Botero is an Associate Professor in information and communication sciences at the Université Paris-Panthéon-Assas and a researcher at Carism, France. As a discourse analyst and semiotician, her research focuses on the mediatization of

1 French Society for Information and Communication Sciences.

2 For more information and recent publications, see: www.allardhuver.fr and www.cv.archives-ouvertes.fr/francois-allard-huver.

ecological issues in France, both in terms of the formal features of these discourses (romanticism, use of metaphors) and public issues (programmed obsolescence, air pollution, pesticides). She has also worked on digital practices related to health and healthcare (rare dermatological conditions, continuation of pregnancy and neonatal palliative care). Her most recent publications are *Influenceurs et influenceuses santé*[3] and *Pollution atmosphérique à la une : visibilité médiatique d'un problème environnemental*[4].

Hélène Ledouble

Hélène Ledouble is an Associate Professor in applied linguistics at the Université de Toulon, France, and a researcher at the Babel laboratory. She works on popular science publications dealing with environmental issues, and is particularly interested in the field of agroecology. Her most recent publications are dedicated to the media coverage of natural plant protection mechanisms (biocontrol, biological control and biopesticides) in the French and English daily press[5].

Authors

Estera Badau

Estera Badau is an Associate Professor in information and communication sciences at the CIMEOS laboratory at the Université de Bourgogne (Communications, media coverage, organizations, knowledge), France. Since completing her doctorate, her research has focused on the links between health and food. After her CIFRE thesis on the links between antibiotic resistance and food, she joined the CIMEOS laboratory, where she is currently leading a research project on thyroid diseases. Her most recent publications are *Médiatisation des liens entre l'usage alimentaire du sel et la santé dans le quotidien Le Monde*[6] and *L'alimentation à l'épreuve du risque et de la controverse*[7].

---

3 Botero, N. (2022). Influenceurs et influenceuses santé. In *Études de communication*, Sedda, P. and Hernandez Orellana, M. (eds), 58.
4 Botero, N. (2021). Pollution atmosphérique à la une : visibilité médiatique d'un problème environnemental. *Revue Française des Sciences de l'Information et de la Communication*, 21.
5 Ledouble, H. (2024). *Popularizing Science: The Complex Terminological Interactions between Scientific and Press Discourses within the Field of Agroecology*. ISTE Ltd, London, and John Wiley & Sons, New York.
6 Badau, E. et al. (in press). Médiatisation des liens entre l'usage alimentaire du sel et la santé dans le quotidien *Le Monde*. *Le Temps des médias*, 41.
7 Badau, E. and Hugol-Gential, C. (2023). L'alimentation à l'épreuve du risque et de la controverse. *Manifeste du réseau AGAP*.

Carole Barthélémy

Carole Barthélémy is a sociologist at Aix-Marseille Université (Population Environment Development Laboratory). She is involved in environmental sociology, working on environmental conflicts and mobilization and on pollution in urban and rural areas. Since 2020, she has coordinated the SHS-pesticides network with Eve-Bureau Point.

José Ramón Bertomeu Sánchez

José Ramón Bertomeu Sánchez is a professor of the history of science at the University of Valencia and a member of the Institut Interuniversitari López Piñero (Spain). His research focuses on the history of forensic medicine and toxic products in France and Spain in the 19th and 20th centuries. He is the author of *Entre el fiscal y el verdugo*[8], a biography of Matthieu Orfila (1787–1853), a renowned Spanish toxicologist. His latest book is *Tóxicos: Pasado y Presente*[9]. His current research project focuses on the social and cultural history of pesticides in 20th-century Spain[10].

Antoine Blanchard

Antoine Blanchard holds a degree in agricultural engineering and a master's degree in the social studies of science and technology. His personal and professional career has taken several directions. His first focus is on digital transformations in the academic and research field: he has been working on these issues at the University of Bordeaux, France, since 2014, with a break between 2020 and 2023 within the Datactivist cooperative society. His second focus is a personal and associative commitment to science-society issues; after co-founding and chairing the Café des sciences community of web popularizers, he joined the board of directors of the Traces association. Last but not least, he holds an interest in environmental issues, particularly in relation to agriculture. He is a freelance researcher on these topics, drawing on approaches from information and communication sciences, digital humanities, and social studies of science and technology.

Eve Bureau-Point

Eve Bureau-Point is an anthropologist at the French National Center for Scientific Research (Centre Norbert Elias, Marseille). She conducts research in

8 Bertomeu, J.R. (2019). *Entre el fiscal y el verdugo*. PUV, Valencia.
9 Bertomeu, J.R. (2021). *Tóxicos: Pasado y Presente*. Icaria, Barcelona.
10 For a list of his publications, see: www.orcid.org/0000-0003-2040-4507.

France and Cambodia on the social life of pesticides (production, market, regulation, uses, waste and residue management). At various stages of her career, she has studied the social construction of environmental health problems. Since 2020, she has coordinated the SHS-pesticides network with Carole Barthélémy.

Louis Galey

Louis Galey is a lecturer in ergonomics at the Université Paris Nanterre, France and a member of the Travail, ergonomie, orientation et organisations (TE2O) team within the Laboratoire parisien de psychologie sociale (LAPPS). He took part in the ARC-CMR project as a member of the EPICENE (Epidemiology of Cancers and Environmental Exposure) team (INSERM, Université de Bordeaux). His doctoral thesis focused on the development of a method for "understanding nanoparticle exposure situations by integrating work activity into the measurement process" in order to build prevention. His postdoctorate at the Centre de recherche sur le travail et le développement (CRTD, CNAM) focused on the activities of social partners in the context of digital transformations.

Alain Garrigou

Alain Garrigou is a professor of ergonomics in INSERM's EPICENE team, and the vice-president in charge of quality of life and health at work at the Université de Bordeaux. His doctoral thesis, supported in 1992 at the CNAM, focused on worker participation in the design of the Figaro printing works. He carries on the legacy of ergonomics pioneers such as Alain Wisner, Catherine Teiger and Antoine Laville, both conceptually and methodologically, as well as the political role of ergonomics research in responding to the social and technological challenges put forward by studies and its changes. For over ten years, he has contributed to the development of ergotoxicology, a transdisciplinary approach integrating ergonomics, public health, toxicology, anthropology and law, with the aim of contributing to the prevention of exposure to substances which can cause cancer.

Fabienne Goutille

Fabienne Goutille is a researcher-speaker in HSS, attached to INRAE's ETTIS (Environment, Territories in Transition, Infrastructures and Societies) research unit. She took part in the ARC-CMR project as a member of the EPICENE team at INSERM (Université de Bordeaux, France). Her doctoral thesis in ergonomics deals with the construction of pesticide risk prevention, and addresses the issue of how farmers' concerns can be taken into account in occupational health policies through extended research communities. The aim of her current work is to support individuals who are working and to make visible and address what challenges them by contributing to the development of personal and collective agency, particularly through the proposal of methods for shared analysis of work or exposures based on popular metrology and developmental ergotoxicology.

Annie Martin

Annie Martin holds a doctorate in private law and is a research fellow at the CNRS Societies, Stakeholders and Governments in Europe. She has a background in private international law and international trade law. Her publications focus on economic law and space law. More recently, her research has focused on conflicts of interest in the field of pharmaceuticals, European pesticide regulation, and the dissemination of standards between international organizations in the chemical sector. She is the author of several book chapters, including "Managing conflicts of interests at the European Medicines Agency. Success or weakness of the soft law tools?"[11] and "The limits to access to information on risks concerning pesticides"[12].

Clémence Rambaud

Clémence Rambaud, a labor lawyer, took part in the ARC-CMR project in 2015 as part of INSERM's EPICENE team.

Jan Smolinski

Jan Smolinski holds a doctorate in sociology, specializing in the sociology of uses, markets and the digital environment, using pragmatic methods. His research ranges from the design of innovations to their assessment, and examines how digital technologies transform user experiences. Sectors include the food industry, mechanical engineering training, tourism, mobile marketing and cultural mediation. As a postdoctoral fellow in the SAGE (Societies, Actors, Government in Europe) laboratory at the University of Strasbourg, France, he is currently involved in the NA'Stras (digital tools for healthy and sustainable food in Strasbourg and the

11 Martin, A. (2021). Managing conflicts of interests at the European Medicines Agency. Success or weakness of the soft law tools? In *Conflict of Interest and Medicine Knowledge, Practices and Mobilizations*, Hauray, B. et al. (eds). Routledge, London.

12 Martin, A. (2017). The limits to access to information on risks concerning pesticides. In *Governance and Perceptions of Hazardous Activities: A Franco-German and European Approach*, Kresse, B. and Lambert, E. (eds). University of Hagen, Hagen.

Bas-Rhin region) and Phyt'Info (digital tools for pesticide reduction) projects. His most recent publications are entitled *Des dispositifs numériques d'aide aux choix alimentaires aux dispositifs des jugements : quelle régulation de l'information des consommateurs?*[13], *Un musée qui conjugue les temps composes*[14] and *How can the use of a mobile application change the course of a sightseeing tour?*[15].

Laurence Thery

Laurence Thery is the Director of Aract Hauts-de-France (Agence régionale d'amélioration des conditions de travail), and holds a master's degree in sociology from Sciences Po Paris. She coordinated the ARC-CMR project with Alain Garrigou in 2015.

Albin Wagener

Albin Wagener is Professor in discourse and communication analysis at the School of Social Sciences at the Catholic University of Lille. Working in the ETHICS research lab, he specifically works on digital, social and environmental discourse in the public, media and political spheres. He specializes in communication issues within social networks. He is the author of *Blablabla : en finir avec le bavardage climatique*[16], *Mèmologie : théorie postdigitale des mèmes*[17], *Ecoarchie*[18] and *Discours et système*[19]. He has also written a study on representations and perceptions linked to climate issues in France, during Emmanuel Macron's first five years in office (2017–2020)[20].

13 Smolinski, J. and Lambert, E. (in press). Des dispositifs numériques d'aide aux choix alimentaires aux dispositifs des jugements : quelle régulation de l'information des consommateurs ? *Revue interdisciplinaire d'études juridiques*.

14 Smolinski, J. (2021). Un musée qui conjugue les temps composés. *Antiquités nationales*, 50–51.

15 Smolinski, J. and Calvignac, C. (2019). How can the use of a mobile application change the course of a sightseeing tour? *Tourist Studies*.

16 Wagner, A. (2023). *Blablabla : en finir avec le bavardage climatique*. Éditions Le Robert, Paris.

17 Wagner, A. (2022). *Mèmologie : théorie postdigitale des mèmes*. Éditions de l'Université de Grenoble-Alpes, Grenoble.

18 Wagner, A. (2021). *Ecoarchie*. Éditions du Croquant, Vulaines-sur-Seine.

19 Wagner, A. (2019). *Discours et système*. Peter Lang, Lausanne.

20 See: www.sysdiscours.hypotheses.org.

Foreword

With the growing power of questioning, social mobilization and lawsuits brought against industries, and also with the increase in public policy systems with reduction objectives, pesticides have become a concerning matter, shaking up the social, economic and political spheres. Researchers in the humanities and social sciences (HSS), attuned to societal changes, have become increasingly involved in these issues. Up until the end of the 20th century, pesticides were rarely the subject of studies in the HSS in their own right. However, since the 2000s, a field of study has been progressively emerging in French academia, with numerous studies, teams and researchers documenting the controversies raised by the production, regulation and use of pesticides[1]. It was against this backdrop of expanding work in the social sciences and humanities that a network was set up in February 2020. Coordinated by Eve Bureau-Point and Carole Barthélémy, it had a view to better identify the scientific community on the subject, the diversity of work in progress, and link people with their knowledge on the subject.

The network's activities focused on organizing a series of study days (annual or biannual) and managing a mailing list designed to facilitate the flow of information concerning HSS work on pesticides (events, publications, calls for projects, etc.). To date, 120 people have subscribed: an almost equal number of men and women, 50 researchers, around 20 teacher-researchers, and 40 doctoral and postdoctoral students, underlining the interest of the subject for young researchers. Around 50 people work for EPSTs, mainly INRAE, while the others work in joint research units. Sociology (37 people) and anthropology (18 people) are the most represented disciplines. Researchers in agronomy (11) and life sciences (10) have also subscribed, underlining the network's appeal to colleagues outside the HSS field.

---

1 Bureau-Point, E. and Temple, L. (2022). La recherche en sciences humaines et sociales sur l'objet pesticide dans le cadre académique français : état des lieux et perspectives. *VertigO – la revue électronique en sciences de l'environnement*, 22, 2.

Economics (11), geography (7) and history (5) are the other main disciplines represented. In addition to facilitating exchanges within the pesticide research, this list is proving to be a very useful way of linking researchers with public policy or civil society players. They can also be used to meet a variety of social demands (such as finding speakers for public debates, improving the research-public policy interface, etc.). They also have several objectives during the study days: to deepen the angles of analysis in HSS on the "pesticides" matter, to reinforce interdisciplinarity (HSS/environmental sciences/medical sciences interactions) and to improve the link between science/society (impact of research in society, research systems and knowledge sharing). On each day, a moment of collective reflection is devoted to the network's coordination and the choice of themes to be addressed on future days. Participants propose new topics, and an organizing committee is set up with the network's initiators and theme leaders. Three study days were thus organized in 2020, 2021 and 2022, each of which was the subject of a publication (a thematic issue in the *VertigO*[2] journal, an article for the "Vie de la recherche" section of the *Natures, sciences et sociétés*[3] journal, and a collective work published by OCTARES)[4]. The fourth study-day event was held in Paris in March 2024, on the theme of pesticide industries.

Other events were organized in parallel with those of the network, such as the "*Pesticides : dialogues pluridisciplinaires en sciences humaines et sociales*" (Pesticides: multidisciplinary dialogues in the humanities and social sciences) study days in Dijon in October 2021, which led to the publication of this collective work. Organized by Nataly Botero, Hélène Ledouble and François Allard-Huver, as well as laboratories specializing in communication and media issues (CIMEOS, CREM, BABEL), these events have provided an opportunity to approach pesticides from the original perspective of linguistics, communication and interdisciplinarity. Case studies from sociology, ergonomics and economics were also presented on other aspects (prevention, public policy, farmer/riparian relations, etc.). The two-day event brought together around 30 participants, who specifically examined the discursive and argumentative activity surrounding pesticides, scientific and communication practices, legal initiatives and court proceedings, as well as productions from the cultural industries. These events were unique in that they brought together academic researchers, independent researchers and activists (crop reapers). Each of the conference contributors addressed these diverse issues from the perspective of their own discipline. Interdisciplinarity was a rare feature of the contributors' research. As

2 Bureau-Point, E. et al. (2021). Les mondes agricoles face au problème des pesticides. Compromis, ajustements et négociations. Introduction au dossier. *VertigO – la revue électronique en sciences de l'environnement*, 21, 3.

3 Bureau-Point, E. et al. (2022). Focus sur les deuxièmes journées d'études du réseau sciences humaines et sociales/pesticides. *Natures, sciences, sociétés*, 30(1), 82–88.

4 See: https://www.octares.com/accueil/306-exposition-aux-pesticides-ce-quen-disent-les-sciences-humaines-et-sociales.html.

the title of this book suggests, the focus was on multidisciplinary. Interdisciplinarity, which implies a real co-construction of research from different disciplines, was ultimately not very frequent in the research schemes of the participants over these few days. Its modalities, benefits and limits can be analyzed in a more specific framework, yet to be determined.

Eve BUREAU-POINT
Centre Norbert-Elias, CNRS
Aix-Marseille Université
France

Carole BARTHÉLÉMY
Laboratoire Population
Environnement Développement
Aix-Marseille Université
France

Introduction

This book presents the work of researchers in the humanities and social sciences (SHS), presented at a conference held at the University of Burgundy in Dijon on October 21 and 22, 2021. The aim of this scientific event was to provide an overview of contemporary research on pesticides in the humanities, as well as to encourage multidisciplinary and interdisciplinary approaches on the subject.

Conceived and organized by researchers from the fields of information and communication science and linguistics, this conference outlined insufficient research in these disciplines. Indeed, the problem of pesticides seems to have been little explored in its communication, language and lexical aspects: a few articles were produced on the media coverage of pesticides in the written press (Ledouble 2020; Botero 2021) or on the controversial aspects of the subject. (Allard-Huver 2021). However, this issue was already debated by numerous geographers, sociologists, ergonomists, anthropologists and historians, which the conference brought together. Some were members of the SHS–Pesticides network, whose work reflects both a growing interest and a change in perspective in the SHS. While for much of the 20th century, pesticides were seen as a vector for agricultural modernization, a turning point has been reached in recent years: pesticides are increasingly being studied as problematic and controversial technologies (Galochet et al. 2008; Roussary et al. 2013; Aulagnier and Goulet 2017; Chateauraynaud and Debaz 2017; Chlous et al. 2017; Catellani et al. 2019; Foucart 2019; Jouzel 2019; Lambert 2020; Bureau-Point et al. 2022). The emergence of this research group and questions concerning the circulation of pesticide-related information in the public sphere reflect a deeper dynamic linked to environmental social sciences. Indeed, while the contribution of life sciences is essential to understanding and highlighting the issues surrounding the use of pesticides, so is the contribution of the SHS.

Introduction written by Nataly BOTERO, Hélène LEDOUBLE and François ALLARD-HUVER.

Our initial aim is to contribute to the emergence of cross-disciplinarity and the transfer of methods specific to interdisciplinarity, which has become necessary to understand the complexity of environmental issues (Jollivet 2008). Convinced of the richness that dialogues, confrontations and debates between different scientific disciplines can bring, such interdisciplinarity has proven difficult to implement and remains a work in progress on this subject, as on others. There are numerous barriers: the need for scientific acculturation to other disciplines; the identification of objects and the fields in between; the social organization of research (particularly in France, where disciplines have differentiated perimeters and are strongly framed by national bodies); the valorization of work in higher education and research; etc. The research presented in this book is therefore more of a multidisciplinary approach, which is nonetheless proving to be a fruitful scientific approach to the problems caused by pesticide use, and suggests avenues for further reflection.

As a result of our interest in discursive and linguistic aspects, this book pays particular attention to the ways in which the object of study is named, what it refers to and what it produces in terms of risks and benefits. Indeed, the act of naming "is less about designating fragments of reality than conveying the speakers' social experience"[1] (Branca Rosoff 2007, p. 14). As this social experience is not devoid of interest, the words used to refer to pesticides are conflicting and competitive. On the one hand, industries, trade unions and public authorities favor relatively established names such as "phytosanitary products" or "phytopharmaceuticals", recalling the need for plant protection, implicitly suggesting the threat imposed by "crop enemies", "pests" and "weeds". These products are thus often presented as unavoidable for agricultural production, food sovereignty and competitiveness. As such, these names can be used in communication strategies aimed at presenting these products in a relatively neutral way, in contrast to current debates on the issues they raise. On the other hand, the names used by associations and professionals with alternative practices, such as "agro-toxic", "biocide" and even "pesticide", have a more conflictual and accusatory impact. We are therefore faced with the same reference, but with a lexicalization which conveys opposite values: while the former are focused on plant protection, the latter evoke their potential to destroy biodiversity.

Historicizing and politicizing pesticide use

Crop protection has been documented since antiquity, with the use of sulfur, copper and arsenic. From the 1960s onwards, agricultural production began to modernize, abandoning the production methods of agrarian societies and adapting to Fordist capitalism. This period saw a series of technological innovations that

1 Author's translation.

enabled unprecedented increases in yields: mechanization, irrigation, monocultures and synthetic pesticides (Deléage 2019). However, this green revolution was achieved "at the cost of serious environmental consequences" (Gisclard 2020, p. 15). Biologists in the United States became interested in these effects, as witnessed by Rachel Carson's *Silent Spring* in 1962. At the same time, toxicologists set out to understand the consequences of pesticide use on human health. These studies were carried out thanks to public pressure, exerted by representatives of immigrant farm workers, who were particularly exposed (Jouzel 2019). With both a cognitive and a moral dimension, pesticide use has rapidly become a public problem in this country. From a cognitive point of view, a production of knowledge began to unfold, revealing facts and figures related to health consequences. Morally speaking, the highly problematic nature of the problem called for its resolution (Gusfield and Cefaï 2009, p. 9).

Historians and sociologists of science have identified three periods corresponding to modes of governance, linked to the widespread toxification of ecosystems and organisms (of which pesticides are just one manifestation). The first period is "government by control" (from the end of World War II to the end of the 1960s), in which pollution was seen as something that could be contained, circumscribed and limited. The second period is "government by risk" (from 1970 to 1990), in which the possibility of damage from pollution was accepted, but this damage remained manageable. The third period is "government by adaptation" (since the 1990s), characterized by the organization of a contaminated world that has become impossible to properly manage. The challenge is no longer to limit it, but to live with it, reflecting a shift in the paradigm of negative externalities, as public authorities disengage in favor of individuals, who are forced to manage their own exposure (Boudia and Jas 2019).

In Europe, challenging the dominant agricultural model only took place in the 1990s, placing farmers between the imperative of productivity and the expectations of civil society (Gisclard 2020), and also reflecting the complex position of regulators and institutions in charge of risk assessment and management. In France, large-scale public measures began with the Grenelle de l'environnement (political environmental forum), launched under the Sarkozy government in 2007. One of the working groups was mandated to reduce "the use of phytopharmaceutical products by 50% within ten years, if possible" (Ministère de l'Agriculture et de l'Alimentation 2020), giving rise to the Écophyto program. Two opposing perspectives clashed within this group: on the one hand, advocates of a systemic vision of agronomy, arguing for the profound transformation of agricultural practices; on the other hand, actors in favor of the substitution of the most dangerous pesticides (Aulagnier and Goulet 2017). This second vision was the one that prevailed from 2012 onwards, and which currently remains dominant in the Écophyto II plan, whose objective has been postponed to 2025. There are at least two reasons for the failure of the systemic vision: firstly, the obligation imposed by the political world to achieve results in the short term; secondly, the reluctance of those working in the field to embrace agri-environmental innovations, who perceived these experiments as risky (Roussary et al. 2013, p. 76).

Controversial molecules, disputed pesticides

Following the ban on domestic and urban use of pesticides in 2014, one of the world's most widely used molecules (glyphosate) was classified as a probable carcinogen by the International Agency for Research on Cancer (IARC) in 2015[2]. This classification is highly controversial, with national agencies such as ANSES[3] in France and the EPA[4] in the United States disagreeing. At stake is the opposition between a "microscopic vision" of a toxicological nature, looking at effects substance by substance, and a "macroscopic vision" carried by epidemiology, looking at long-term effects on health (Jouzel 2019; Lambert 2020).

Despite this classification, the authorization of glyphosate was extended in November 2023 by the European Union for a further 10 years, until 2033. Some authors consider that this decision "was produced and calibrated according to preexisting political and economic interests" (Pénet 2019, p. 98), not scientific knowledge. This is not a matter of a lack of knowledge, but of "strategic ignorance", leading to the dismissal of research that has already been carried out, or to the demonstration of the safety of controversial molecules. While the call for ever more research can be positive, it can also induce "the misleading idea that current knowledge is insufficient to take action" (Foucart 2021, p. 151).

The use of pesticides is currently the subject of intense public debate in the media, politics and associations. On the media front, recent studies have concluded that simplifying the distinction between "good" and "bad" pesticides (biopesticides versus chemical pesticides), as well as ambiguous terminology, prevents the general public from grasping these complex issues (Ledouble 2020). On the political front, the derogation granted in 2020 to neonicotinoids, the so-called "bee-killer" pesticides, has been the subject of considerable controversy. Clashing opinions from associations and citizens' movements are rising up: by making this issue their own, they are turning it from a strictly agricultural issue into a societal one.

In the first quarter of 2023 alone, we discovered the extent of surface and groundwater pollution caused by chlorothalonil metabolites (despite it being banned

---

2 See: https://www.iarc.who.int/

3 French National agency for food, environment and work security (https://www.anses.fr/fr)

4 US Environment Protection Agency (https://www.epa.gov/)

in 2019); the Court of Justice of the European Union banned derogations for neonicotinoids; and the chlordecone trial in Martinique and Guadeloupe was finally dismissed. On the subject of chlordecone, this decision comes after many twists and turns: solutions to replace one product with others, derogations followed by a ban with no immediate effect, lack of monitoring and expertise on contamination, and recognition as a victim aimed solely at occupational cancers. These repeated failures have led some authors to bring up decisions based on a colonial vision of the overseas territories (Le Moal and Pierre-Charles 2022).

While damage to human health is a serious matter, damage to ecosystems and biodiversity is just as serious. The massive disappearance of insects and birds made the headlines in several newspapers during the same period, with these issues also being addressed by NGOs through the "justice for the living world" legal action. The negative consequences of pesticide use are numerous, protean and systemic (public health, water, air and soil pollution, threats to biodiversity), so much so that it would not be wrong to view them as a "crisis" (Baxerres et al. 2021).

Pesticides through the humanities and social sciences prism: the three phases of the book

This book is divided into three parts, each comprising two or three chapters. The first reflects on the dynamics of pesticide reduction in France, its practices and trajectories. The second looks at international approaches to pesticide use, while the third focuses on media, institutional and digital discourses on pesticides.

In the first part of this book, the issue of reducing pesticide use is addressed from ergotoxicological and sociological perspectives, as well as from the experience of a member of an association working to reduce or even ban the use of these products.

The study entitled "Ergotoxicology Applications to Characterize Pesticide Exposures in Real Work"[5], by Fabienne Goutille and a team of multidisciplinary researchers (ergotoxicology, ergonomics, law and psychology), offers a review and reflections on the ergotoxicological approach. Based on two projects carried out in the agricultural sector, the authors show how ergotoxicology can be used to understand pesticide exposure and help reduce it, by highlighting the determinants of exposure. Ergotoxicology will thus help working people to understand the harmfulness of their work environment, and to transform it through the way they experience their own working conditions.

5 Original French title: "Applications de l'ergotoxicologie pour caractériser les expositions aux pesticides dans le travail reel".

Jan Smolinski, a sociology researcher at the University of Strasbourg, presents a chapter entitled “Thinking about Pesticides in Terms of a ‘Socio-technical Lock-in’ of Information”[6]. According to the author, the context of “tense” food markets and “sensitive communication” linked to the use of the term “pesticides” invites us to consider the ways in which mentions or claims related to the use of phytosanitary products are expressed in the production process of food products. This chapter proposes a specification of this market context and examines the conditions for defining food quality, based on the exemplary co-construction of two sociotechnical consumer information systems that mention the term “pesticides”. Based on this observation, hypotheses are formulated with a view to extracting ways of unlocking or circumventing the constraints imposed by a “concerned” market.

This first part closes with an interview with Dominique Masset, an activist, member of the *Faucheurs Volontaires* collective, initiator and co-chairman of the Glyphosate Campaign and co-chairman of the *Secrets toxiques* campaign. In this interview, conducted by Nataly Botero, Hélène Ledouble and François Allard-Huver and entitled “Activist Measures and Legal Levers: An Interview with Dominique Masset”[7], the interviewee looks back at the origins of his activism, his motivations and the different modalities of environmental struggles (legal recourse, communication, media relations). This exchange details a reflexive metadiscourse from associative actors on how to name their causes, how to communicate appropriately to different audiences, and how to encourage understanding of the issues and garner commitment from everyone. Dominique Masset insists on the distinction between farmers and the system in which they are caught, pointing in particular to the responsibilities of an agricultural production system that is solely driven by the pursuit for financial profit, which harms both its workers and ecosystems.

The second part presents two chapters based on an international, legal, historical and socio-economic perspective. This section opens with a contribution by Annie Martin, a CNRS research fellow, entitled “The Globalization of Regulatory Science on Pesticides: History and Effects on European Law”[8]. This chapter offers a legal and historical perspective on the globalization of regulatory science on pesticides as controversial objects. It invites us to question the history of technical norms by showing the discrepancy between the regulations that make the marketing of pesticides conditional on the production of scientific proof that this chemical object does not have unacceptable effects on the environment and health, and another

6 Original French title: “Penser les pesticides au regard d’un ‘verrouillage sociotechnique’ informnel”.
7 Original French title: “Trajectoires militantes et leviers juridiques”.
8 Original French title: “La circulation des méthodes de production des connaissances sur les pesticides de l’OCDE vers l’Union européenne: histoire et effets”.

science, produced outside of any standard perspective, invites us to question the history of this technical standardization. In the first part, this study focuses on the ideas and standard instruments developed and disseminated since the early 1970s by a major player in the globalization of pesticide regulatory science, the Organisation for Economic Co-operation and Development (OECD). In the second part, the author shows that OECD regulatory science has flowed into European law, and that this contributes to ignorance about the harmfulness of pesticides.

The second contribution in this section is by José Ramón Bertomeu Sánchez, a historian at the University of Valencia (Spain), entitled "Fighting the Colorado Potato Beetle in Francoist Spain (1939–1953)"[9]. This text develops a historical and political perspective of the massive introduction of pesticides into Spanish agriculture in the 1940s. Conceived as the preferred means of combating pests (in particular the Colorado beetle), this approach marginalized other methods such as biological control (which was undergoing significant development in the first half of the 20th century). The author explains this by the autarky policies of the Franco government, which developed a set of measures encouraging the use of arsenic pesticides. He highlights the significant role played by agricultural engineers, a professional body that articulated agrarian modernization projects with the policies of the authoritarian regime. Focusing on the province of Burgos, an analysis is made of communication campaigns aimed at overcoming farmers' resistance. The arrival of DDT, which was authorized and widely used, took place against a backdrop of numerous decrees, resulting in a legal architecture that favored the deployment and use of pesticides, while glossing over the toxic risks for populations and ecosystems.

The third and final part of this book adopts a discursive and communicative perspective, focusing on media productions (particularly the written press), professional productions (technical documents, trade press) and digital productions (comments on social networks). For example, Estera Badau, an associate professor in communication studies, has written a chapter entitled "From Pesticides to Thyroid Diseases: Media Coverage of a Nameless Problem"[10]. This diachronic study presents the initial results of an ongoing research project (ThyroSIC), aimed at studying the publicization of thyroid disease in France. It specifically focuses on media coverage of the links between pesticides and thyroid disease, based on a corpus of articles published by the daily French newspaper *Le Monde*. Scientific studies showing that certain pesticides are endocrine disruptors have been covered by the media, with these same studies also being taken up by public institutions. The analysis shows a two-phase media coverage: before 2013, a few published articles mainly reported on the link between pesticide use and various types of cancer, including thyroid cancer.

---

9 Original French title: "La lutte contre le doryphore dans l'Espagne de Franco (1939-1953)".

10 Original French title: "Des pesticides aux maladies de la thyroïde : médiatisation d'un problème sans nom".

After 2013, scientific knowledge on endocrine disruptors became more numerous and precise, revealing numerous ramifications, from the environment to food and health.

The penultimate chapter of this book is written by Antoine Blanchard, a graduate agronomist with a master's degree in the social studies of science and technology. It is entitled "Discursive Strategies of a Sociotechnical Network: The Case of Plant Resistance Inducers (PRIs)"[11], and its main question concerns the way in which plant resistance inducers have served the promises of this new phytosanitary paradigm over a decade (1997–2007), while setting them apart from existing solutions. The French acronym "SDN" is analyzed using both a quantitative approach to content analysis and a qualitative approach drawn from linguistics. The author proposes a review of the discursive strategy of SDNs in five singular communicative spaces (scientific literature, technical and commercial documentation, the trade press, the general public press, and the scientific and technical popularization press). He then compares this discursive strategy with that of biopesticides. His work brings to light a kaleidoscopic image of the SDN sociotechnical network, around a common repertoire, creating an "SDN world" in which we are called to come and live.

Proposed by Albin Wagener, a discourse analyst and specialist in environmental issues, the final text in this collective work is entitled "Circulation of Discourses and Counter-discourses about Pesticides on Social Networks"[12]. The author points out that for several decades now, the dangerousness of pesticides has been making media-influenced incursions into public debate. Underpinned by a large number of studies and legal positions, the complexity of the subject has led to a massive production of discourse and counter-discourse. He points out that discourses and counter-discourses about pesticides vary, because from neonicotinoids to glyphosate, public media controversies have given rise to a wide variety of narratives. His chapter focuses on analyzing the conversations taking place in comments on social networks. To this end, the author has built up a digital corpus from social networks in order to access representations within discourses, taking into account the specificities of environmental and ecology-related discourses. This corpus is analyzed using lexicometric analysis, with a view to providing a topography of representations and their positioning in relation to pesticide-related social issues.

11 Original French title: "Stratégies discursives d'un réseau sociotechnique : le cas des stimulateurs des défenses naturelles des plantes (SDN)".

12 Original French title: "Circulation de discours et contre-discours à propos des pesticides sur les réseaux sociaux".

References

Allard-Huver, F. (2021). Ce que les SIC font aux controverses environnementales, ce que les controverses environnementales font aux SIC. *Revue française des sciences de l'information et de la communication*, 21. doi: 10.4000/rfsic.10215.

Aulagnier, A. and Goulet, F. (2017). Des technologies controversées et de leurs alternatives. Le cas des pesticides agricoles en France. *Sociologie du travail*, 59(3). doi: 10.4000/sdt.840.

Baxerres, C., Dussy, D., Musso, S. (2021). Le vivant face aux "crises" sanitaires. *Anthropologie & santé. Revue internationale francophone d'anthropologie de la santé*, 22 [Online]. Available at: https://journals.openedition.org/anthropologiesante/9735 [Accessed 4 May 2023].

Botero, N. (2021). Soustraire l'alimentation du débat sur les pesticides : traitement médiatique d'un problème en une. In *Qu'est-ce que l'on mange ? Les savoirs alimentaires à l'aune des Sciences de l'Information et de la Communication*, Hugol-Gential, C. and Badau, E. (eds). Éditions Universitaires de Dijon, Dijon [Online]. Available at: https://hal.archives-ouvertes.fr/hal-03548223 [Accessed 4 May 2023].

Boudia, S. and Jas, N. (2019). *Gouverner un monde toxique*. Editions Quae, Versailles.

Branca Rosoff, S. (2007). *L'acte de nommer. Une dynamique entre langue et discours*. Presses Sorbonne Nouvelle, Paris.

Bureau-Point, È., Aulagnier, A., Barthélémy, C., El Kotni, M., Goulet, F., Hunsmann, M., Jas, N., Temple, L. (2022). Les pesticides au prisme des sciences humaines et sociales. Focus sur les deuxièmes journées d'études du réseau SHS-Pesticides. *Natures sciences sociétés*, 30(1), 82–88. doi: 10.1051/nss/2022024.

Carson, R. (2002). *Silent Spring*. Houghton Mifflin, Boston.

Catellani, A., Pascual Espuny, C., Pudens Malibabo, L., Jalenques Vigouroux, B. (2019). Les recherches en communication environnementale. *Communication*, 36(2) [Online]. Available at: http://journals.openedition.org/communication/10559 [Accessed 4 May 2023].

Chateauraynaud, F. and Debaz, J. (2017). *Aux bords de l'irréversible. Sociologie pragmatique des transformations*. Pétra, Paris.

Chlous, F., Dozières, A., Guillaud, D., Legrand, L. (2017). Des recherches participatives dans la production des savoirs liés à l'environnement – Introduction. Foisonnement participatif : des questionnements communs ? *Natures sciences sociétés*, 25(4), 327–335.

Deléage, J.-P. (2019). Une alimentation digne et saine pour tous ! *Écologie & politique*, 59(2), 5–13. doi: 10.3917/ecopo1.059.0005.

Foucart, S. (2019). *Et le monde devint silencieux. Comment l'agrochimie a détruit les insectes*. Éditions du Seuil, Paris.

Galochet, M., Longuepee, J., Morel, V., Petit, O. (eds) (2008). *L'environnement : discours et pratiques interdisciplinaires*. Artois Presses Université, Arras.

Gisclard, M. (2020) Agriculture. In *Dictionnaire critique de l'anthropocène*, Alexandre, F. and Argounès, F. (eds). CNRS Éditions, Paris.

Gusfield, J.R. and Cefaï, D. (2009). *La culture des problèmes publics : l'alcool au volant la production d'un ordre symbolique*. Economica, London.

Jollivet, M. (2008). Préface. In *L'environnement : discours et pratiques interdisciplinaires*, Galochet, M., Longuépée, J., Morel, V., Petit, O. (eds). Artois Presses Université, Arras.

Jouzel, J.-N. (2019). *Pesticides : comment ignorer ce que l'on sait*. Presses de Sciences Po, Paris.

Kleinman, D.L. and Suryanarayanan, S. (2013). Dying bees and the social production of ignorance. *Science, Technology, & Human Values*, 38(4), 492–517. doi: 10.1177/0162243912442575.

Lambert, E. (2020). Le contentieux américain des victimes de l'exposition au glyphosate. *Revue juridique de l'environnement*, HS20, 201–213.

Le Moal, P. and Pierre-Charles, P. (2022). Chlordécone, un crime d'État impuni ? In *Écologies : le vivant et le social*, Boursier, P. and Guimont, C. (eds). La Découverte, Paris.

Ledouble, H. (2020). Term circulation and conceptual instability in the mediation of science: Binary framing of the notions of biological versus chemical pesticides. *Discourse and Communication*, 14(5), 466–488. doi: 10.1177/1750481320917575.

Ministère de l'Agriculture et de l'Alimentation (2020). Le plan Écophyto, qu'est-ce que c'est ? [Online]. Available at: https://agriculture.gouv.fr/le-plan-ecophyto-quest-ce-que-cest [Accessed 4 May 2023].

Pénet, P. (2019). Fake science et ignorance stratégique : retour sur les récentes controverses autour de l'austérité et du glyphosate. *Études de communication*, 53, 85–101.

Roussary, A., Busca, D., Salles, D., Dumont, A., Carpy-Goulard, F. (2013). Pratiques phytosanitaires en agriculture et environnement. Des tensions irréductibles ? *Économie rurale. Agricultures, alimentations, territoires*, 333. doi: 10.4000/economierurale.3804.

1

Ergotoxicology in Action: Understanding Work-Activity Pesticide Exposures

The authors would like to thank all of those who took part in the active research described here, particularly René Baratta, Marie-Hélène Devier, Isabelle Baldi and Pierrick Pasquereau. We would also like to express our gratitude to all of those who, both on and off farms, have contributed to our work on characterizing real-life exposure to pesticides.

1.1. Introduction

This chapter reviews and reflects on the ergotoxicology approach. Based on two projects carried out in the agricultural sector, this chapter shows how ergotoxicology has been used to understand pesticide exposure and help reduce it by highlighting its determinants.

In the first part, the ergotoxicological approach is described in terms of its origins, its objectives and its ability to integrate real work into the characterization of chemical exposure. Two examples of ergotoxicological applications are developed to illustrate the approach. The actions carried out in the workplace are described in detail: from the implementation of metrological tools to the discussion of measurement results in relation to the work activity and its determinants. A summary outlines the results of the two ergotoxicological procedures in relation to preventive action. The role of the people affected by exposure and preventive action

---

Chapter written by Fabienne GOUTILLE, Louis GALEY, Clémence RAMBAUD, Laurence THERY and Alain GARRIGOU.

are discussed in a dialogue between disciplines working to characterize and reduce pesticide exposure.

1.2. Ergotoxicology

In particular, ergotoxicological approaches have highlighted the limits of the dominant models for preventing occupational chemical risks, which are particularly based on the setting of indicative occupational exposure limits (OELs) values derived from toxicological tests, and on the recommendation of individual and collective protective equipment (Garrigou et al. 2008). These models are based on a "decontextualized" vision of work, conceived as a prescribed task rather than a concrete activity. Ergotoxicologists, on the other hand, have shown that a better understanding of chemical hazards can only be achieved by grasping work situations in all their complexity. Observation of the body at work, of its postures, and study of the work environment, are therefore essential for the prevention of chemically-induced occupational illnesses (Jouzel and Dedieu 2011, p. 255).

1.2.1. *Characterizing exposure in real work*

Ergotoxicology (Villatte 1983; Sznelwar 1992; Mohammed-Brahim and Garrigou 2009; Garrigou 2011), a specialized field of ergonomics (Falzon 2004, p. 18), aims to characterize exposures to chemical substances and proposes effective tools and means of prevention, in order to avert health risks to the workers (Galey et al. 2019). Today, it is recognized by the need to integrate elements related to actual work in the analysis of exposures; in other words, by the "need to analyze individuals' exposures by taking practices into account, so as to grasp the elements that combine with one another in real-life situations" (Laurent et al. 2016).

Ergotoxicology is part of "a real work battle" (Duraffourg and Vuillon 2004); in other words, the need to look beyond prescribed work, based on organizational norms and anticipations, and to consider the work as it is performed, and what this performance specifically demands of each person in its various human and social aspects (Daniellou 1997; Fucks and Bourmaud 2011). Alongside experimental toxicological and epidemiological standards which support a macroscopic characterization of occupational exposures, observing real work is complementary to the production of generic data on exposures. The analysis of exposures in work situations can then empirically build up an in-depth characterization of exposures and contribute to the production of specific data, so as to equip risk prevention with a transformative objective.

In an attempt to solve the enigma of exposure and to understand chemical exposure in all its complexity, ergotoxicologists draw on the knowledge of ergonomics and toxicology, coupled with other complementary disciplines (industrial hygiene, metrology, occupational medicine, ethnography, etc.). Part of the approach is aimed at identifying high-risk work situations and qualifying the ways in which people come into contact (Vézina 2001) with sources of danger (occurrence, duration, frequency, etc.). Direct contact (with a chemical and its derivatives) or indirect contact (with a soiled surface) is revealed by means of ergonomic observations, targeted and constructed metrology (Goutille 2022), video exposure monitoring (Galey et al. 2019) and the workers' perceptions of risk (Goutille et al. 2016). The aim is not to demonstrate the dose–effect of a chemical substance, or to establish the link between the use of a substance and its effect on health, but rather to identify the conditions under which exposures are produced, which need to be prevented and changed.

One of the foundations of the practice is thus based on understanding toxic substances and analyzing the behavior of the "substances involved" in work situations (Mohammed-Brahim 2000). Ergotoxicology considers exposure variability as a function of work organization (schedules, processes, raw materials, etc.), operating modes, work tools and the characteristics and dynamics of the people involved. By observing and documenting exposures, several measurements are coupled together to simultaneously assess different types of exposure (e.g. physical and chemical), and to measure their interaction beyond regulatory requirements:

– physiological or biomechanical measurements (heart and respiratory rates, skin temperature, joint angulation, eye strain, effort and force applied when handling materials, etc.) in parallel with the activity performed (postures, gestures, positioning in the workspace, durations or occurrences of actions, movements, flows, communications);

– measurements of chemical concentrations (dust, solvents, volatile organic compounds, gases, fumes, etc.), coupled with the physical characteristics of the working environment (noise, temperature, humidity, air speed, lighting, workstation dimensions, distance from pollutant extraction systems, etc.);

– known toxicological risk discussed in view of the sensory knowledge of working people.

The challenge lies in identifying peaks in exposure (physical effort, contact with soiled surfaces, types of posture, etc.) and concentrations (dust, volatile organic compounds, particles, etc.), the conditions of their origin and the phases of activity to which they correspond (Garrigou 2011).

To develop chemical risk prevention within work organizations, one of the techniques used in ergotoxicology is the simple or crossover self-confrontation interview (Clot 1999; Theureau 2010). This involves offering working people a new context, in which they become external observers of work activity and adopt an analytical posture in the presence of a third party (Judon 2017). This system aims to move from general discourse on work to a more precise verbalization of the nature and motives that guide the various actions (Baratta 1997). This technique calls for activity (Van Belleghem 2015) and enables skills to develop while security is built (Nascimento et al. 2013).

Traces of activity and chemical risk (procedures, graphs, plans, anecdotes as well as filmed sequences of work and measurement results) are circulated between company players to document chemical risk situations. These traces become "intermediate objects of dialogue" (Judon 2017) between those involved in the targeted work situation and those outside the activity, whether internal or external to the company (other employees, occupational physician, family members, designers, researchers, etc.). Complementary characteristics of the activity initially invisible (Béguin 1997) then emerge, providing new resources for understanding the determinants of exposure and taking preventive action. In a number of ergotoxicological interventions, this technique has enabled us to identify prevention practices that manage chemical risks, from which we can build prevention action to complement regulated prevention (Garrigou et al. 2015, 2017; Goutille et al. 2016).

This chapter focuses on the application of the ergotoxicological approach to the characterization of pesticide exposure in agricultural environments. It should be noted that this approach is the result of numerous experiments carried out in various occupational environments exposed to pesticides (Sznelwar 1992; Mohammed-Brahim 1996; Garrigou et al. 2008; Albert 2018; Goutille 2022; Jolly 2022) and other hindrances (asbestos, bitumen fumes, nanoparticles, etc.) as shown in Galey et al. (2020).

1.2.2. *The participation of working people*

Ergotoxicology considers working people as experts on work performance and activity, as well as key players in the understanding and transformation of problematic situations. Given the right knowledge, skills, feelings and burdens, as well as the right tools, support, resources and encouragement, they are best placed to identify and analyze problems, and to develop and implement solutions that are both effective (in reducing risk and improving productivity), desirable and acceptable to the people concerned.

There are many types of participation, including consultative or representative, where users or elected representatives, respectively, express ideas or opinions, and management makes the decisions. Here, however, we are more interested in direct

(Vink et al. 2006) and emancipatory (Goutille and Garrigou 2021) participation, in which working people have an influence over decisions concerning changes in the workplace. This approach aims to give a voice to working people who are ignored by conventional prevention and design approaches (Goutille 2022), and to restore movements (Le Bossé 2012) and collective initiatives for psychological health (Clot and Granger 2019, paragraph 14) among those who are not in a position of power.

The needs of isolated or unrepresented minority groups, and of those with additional needs in the workplace, can be documented through an ergotoxicological approach that feeds into an inclusive and developmental design process. The need to understand exposures as they happen, rather than as they are imagined or as they are regulated, has led ergotoxicologists to recognize the importance and value of co-constructing the characterization and transformation of risk situations with the people who actually experience chemical exposure. This enables ergotoxicologists to have a fuller and broader understanding of how work tasks are performed, how they vary between working people and how tasks can change in response to other system demands and requirements. It should be noted that this approach also enables us to identify the individual and collective ideas and resources that working people have for improving system performance.

The aim of implementing specific systems is designed to enable working people to express and discuss their perceptions and understandings of risks in certain situations, whether they are considered to be embodied expertise (Mohammed-Brahim 2009) or fine-grained empirical knowledge concerning the hazards encountered (Judon 2017). These systems, built on a dialogical framework of expression (in the sense of Callon et al. (2001)), make it possible to initiate a mutual learning process between heterogeneous actors (Béguin 2004). The intermediate objects used (toxicological data sheet, filmed work phases, measurement results, exposure cartography, etc.) support the pivoting points of view and the development of plural thinking for collective action on the determinants of exposure. The subjectivity of the people involved is thus used and elicited, in order to act with subjects and collectives in the conflicts they experience (Clot and Granger 2019), as well as support them in producing knowledge aimed at transforming harmful environments. These activity summoning systems therefore make it possible to bring the real work perspective (Duraffourg and Vuillon 2004) into work design processes, which aim to take care of the worker (Guérin et al. 2021), by getting closer to realities in the field.

1.3. Examples of ergotoxicology applications in agriculture

To illustrate the ergotoxicological approach and its use in characterizing pesticide exposure, we will develop two examples from research and intervention work. Both are based on the French agricultural sector, with the aim of promoting the constructed prevention of pesticide risk, related to the use of phytopharmaceutical products (Goutille 2022).

The examples selected are based on different applications of ergotoxicology. One is a retrospective analysis of pesticide metrology results based on work analysis, while the other is an analysis of pesticide risk situations based on targeted pesticide metrology.

The first example focuses on the visibility of the levels and determinants of pesticide exposure, in the context of the use of personal protective equipment (PPE) for the application of plant protection products. The associated Pestexpo program aimed to characterize the factors of pesticide contamination in field crops and vineyards, by integrating ergotoxicology with field epidemiology (Garrigou 2011; Baldi et al. 2012, 2014).

The second analysis of pesticide risk situations illustrated in the practice of potato thermal fogging is part of the ARC-CMR project (Garrigou et al. 2015). This project, which was implemented within companies of different sizes and in different sectors, aimed to use ergotoxicology to highlight exposures that are barely perceptible, as well as question the conditions under which prevention is built in the face of vague, diffuse and indirect carcinogenic, mutagenic and reprotoxic risks.

1.3.1. *The contribution of ergotoxicology to field epidemiology in the analysis of pesticide contamination among pesticide farmers*

1.3.1.1. *The Pestexpo program*

Measurements of the contamination of French pesticide farmers with tracer pesticides[1] were carried out as part of the Pestexpo program (2000–2006), run by two epidemiology laboratories, GRÉCAN in Caen and the EPICENE-INSERM team at the University of Bordeaux. The Pestexpo program provides algorithms describing pesticide contamination in France's main agricultural contexts. Contamination measurements carried out under actual conditions of pesticide use by farmers have made it possible to describe the circumstances relating to the risks of direct and indirect contamination.

1 The use of tracer pesticides involves measuring one or more pesticides and generalizing the results obtained for all pesticides, while considering the limits of this extrapolation. In the case of Pestexpo, dithiocarbamates and folpel were chosen, as these active ingredients have been widely used in French viticulture over recent decades.

In epidemiological terms, the risk of direct pesticide contamination corresponds to direct contact of the skin, eyes, nose or hair with pesticides. The risk of indirect contamination concerns any contact with a contaminated element, such as equipment, product packaging, plants, soil and surfaces, work equipment, tools and machinery, protective clothing and equipment.

The results of the Pestexpo program have been analyzed retrospectively using an ergotoxicological approach, in order to define the determinants of pesticide contamination among winegrowers who use plant protection products. We present here how ergotoxicology, based on an analysis of real work, was able to highlight the determinants of pesticide contamination among users of plant protection products, and to alert us to the ineffectiveness of the protective coveralls recommended for use. Here, we will take up part of Alain Garrigou's unpublished dissertation (Garrigou 2011).

1.3.1.2. *Methodology for characterizing contaminants and their determinants*

Pesticide contamination was determined during the various operations involved in the use of phytopharmaceutical products. The methodology, derived from industrial hygiene, was adopted in expology and supplemented by activity analysis when interpreting the results for winegrowing.

For vineyard treatment activities in Gironde, 72 observation days were carried out in real-life situations, focusing on the preparation and application of phytosanitary sprays using backpack sprayers (five days) or towed sprayers (67 days). Other observation days focused on the contamination of winegrowing professionals during reentry and harvesting operations.

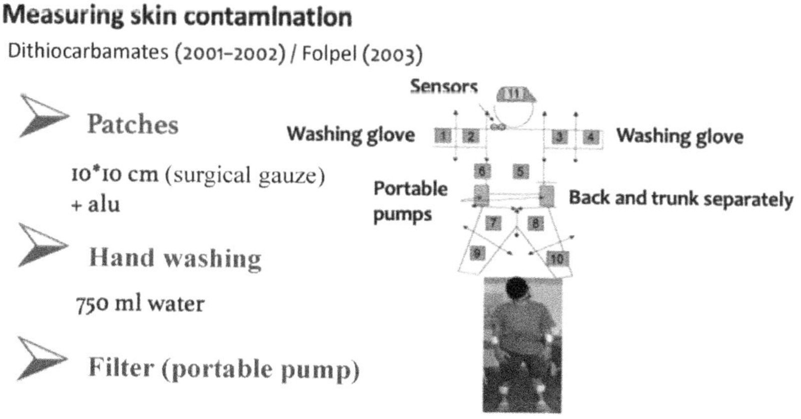

Figure 1.1. *Measuring contamination (Garrigou 2011, p. 65). For a color version of this figure, see www.iste.co.uk/botero/pesticides.zip*

Contamination was measured by analyzing the quantity of phytosanitary product deposited on 10 cm^2 surgical gauze patches. These patches were directly attached to the skin (see Figure 1.1). They were changed between different work operations (preparation, application, cleaning) in order to compare contamination between different phases of activity (see Figure 1.2).

Analyses were also carried out on handwashing water, urine samples and filters to assess the risk of penetration via the respiratory tract. The protocol met the OECD's (1997) recommendations for this type of field study.

During the preparation phases, almost two-thirds of people were protected according to their work habits, slightly more than half for the application and more than half for the cleaning; however, just because the winegrowers wore coveralls, it does not mean that they were protected enough to avoid all contamination, as we will discuss later.

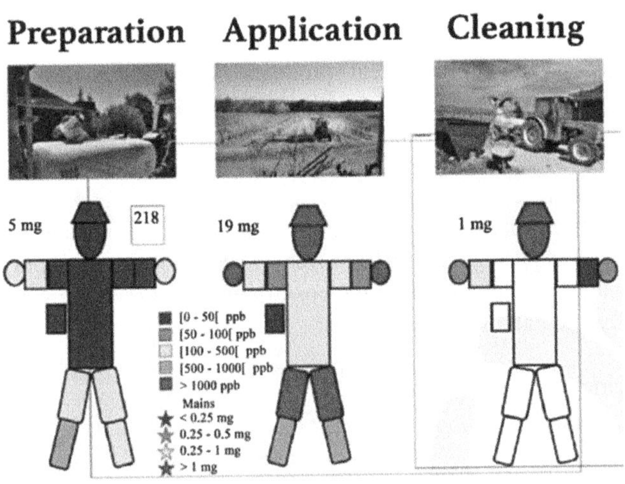

Figure 1.2. *Metrology results (by patches) by activity phase. Adapted from Baldi et al. (2012). For a color version of this figure, see www.iste.co.uk/botero/pesticides.zip*

1.3.1.3. *Results of the Pestexpo contamination program*

According to the results of Pestexpo, pesticide contamination in farming occurs at all stages of the phytopharmaceutical treatment process. Contamination may occur before the products are used, for example, during storage, spray preparation, particularly when products are introduced into the equipment, or as a result of technical hazards (tank overflow, excessive foaming and the formation of clumps).

Contamination has also been identified during the spraying of crops, particularly in the event of incidents (e.g. nozzle clogging) that lead professionals to intervene on contaminated equipment. The Pestexpo results show that contamination may also occur during the cleaning and maintenance of spraying equipment (filters, nozzles, tanks).

Reentry operations in treated plots may also appear to be critical exposure phases. Contamination has been observed when reentering treated crops for other tasks (indirect contamination when handling treated plants). This type of result was behind the introduction of reentry periods in France in 2006.

Pesticide content in the urine of applicators shows that contamination does not depend "on the quantity of plant protection products used or the surface area treated, but on the method of application and the level of protection of the applicator" (Gatignol and Étienne 2010, p. 137).

1.3.1.4. *Ergotoxicology's contribution to pesticide risk prevention*

1.3.1.4.1. Ergotoxicology's contribution to the interpretation of contamination results with or without coveralls

When it comes to chemical risks, and in particular, the risk of pesticide exposure, even though comprehensive prevention approaches have been developed by prevention institutions, it has to be said that the prevention measures that are most often implemented are PPE. From a regulatory perspective, priority must be given to collective protection, but in reality, this is lacking in the field, for a variety of reasons: high cost in relation to possible investments for farmers, technologies that are not always adapted to the specificities of agriculture, etc. Legally, the safety obligation falls to the employer of labor, the farm manager or the company director. This means that they have an obligation toward the result: in the event of exposure and contamination by products that could cause health problems, they could be held responsible.

A survey by the French Ministry of Agriculture (2006) revealed that the recommended protective equipment was rarely worn, which raises questions about the real effectiveness of preventive practices and resources. Several authors had already highlighted the difficulties associated with wearing PPE and the constraints it generates (Baldi et al. 2023). The effectiveness of protective equipment in real-life conditions therefore has major implications in terms of both health and liability, as defined by the French Labor Laws.

By analyzing the data from the 67 observations involving treatment with a tractor and sprayer, we can detail the frequency of wearing PPE as follows:

– 50% of winegrowers did not wear gloves, 40% wore them during one of the two phases of preparation or application (2% in this case) and only 10% for both phases.

– 58% never wore coveralls, 24% during one of the two phases (of which only 4% during application) and 18% during both phases.

– 61% never wore coveralls, 36% wore them for one of the two phases (including 4% for application) and only 3% for both phases.

The results were expressed in milligrams of active ingredient (dithiocarbamates) deposited on the skin (after extrapolation of the patch to the surface of the area under consideration). Figure 1.3 shows that people wearing clothing were more likely to be contaminated than people not wearing clothing.

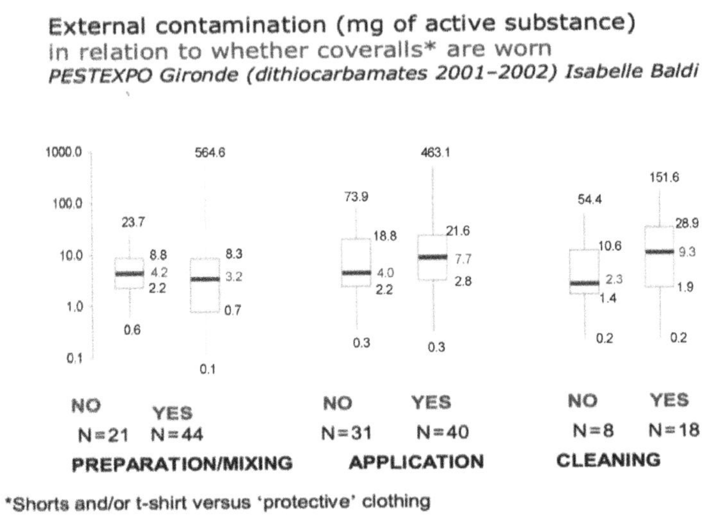

Figure 1.3. *Measuring skin contamination according to whether or not coveralls are worn (Garrigou 2011, p. 90). For a color version of this figure, see www.iste.co.uk/botero/pesticides.zip*

These results have raised eyebrows in the prevention community, since one of the strong focuses of the recommendations is the wearing of personal protective clothing, in particular type 4 coveralls to protect against aerosols (according to NF EN 14 605, type 4 is "protection against liquid chemicals. Equipment providing complete or partial protection of the wearer against liquid chemicals in the form of a spray").

Beyond the possible penetration of chemicals, permeation phenomena have been observed in the laboratory on type 4 coveralls on a molecular scale. A wide range of plant protection products commonly used in agriculture were found to migrate inside the tested coveralls. These results are extremely alarming, as it is likely that sweat generated by physical exertion, which cannot evaporate because it is trapped in the coverall, can promote the penetration of phytopharmaceutical products inside the coverall.

After discussions with coverall manufacturers, it emerged that the coveralls recommended for agriculture and initially developed for industry had not originally been tested against the active ingredients contained in the plant protection products used, including the most common ones (Garrigou 2011). Wearing coveralls could limit exposure during the preparation phase, but would not totally prevent contamination: "during the treatment and cleaning phases, people who wore coveralls were overall more contaminated than those who did not" (Garrigou 2011, p. 90).

The measurement of the protective capabilities of type 4 coveralls revealed shortcomings in the suit's performance under real-life conditions of plant protection product use. These results gave rise to a warning about the unreliability of protective equipment in the use of plant protection products. The contribution of ergotoxicology (analysis of activities and contaminations) to the construction of a collective alert process is detailed by Garrigou (2011, pp. 95–98). It was the comparison of permeation data produced by a manufacturer of plant protection products with those from Pestexpo, discussed from the point of view of real-life work, that highlighted the importance of the problem.

1.3.1.4.2. Explanatory hypotheses for contamination

Following a series of discussions with various experts in the field (the Agricultural Social Security Mutual (MSA) funds, the Institut national de recherche et de sécurité (INRS), the National and European Union of Manufacturers of Plant Protection Products, the Direction générale du travail and the French Ministry of Agriculture), Garrigou et al. (2008, 2011) proposed various hypotheses to explain contamination and its variability according to work contexts. We take up these hypotheses, based on the ergotoxicological approach:

1) Individual and collective expertise of how to be safe, developed and capitalized on by winegrowing professionals over the course of their experience.

2) Organization and preparation of work activities to anticipate hazards.

3) Lack of advice on the use, maintenance and cleaning of protective equipment and materials.

4) Inadequate consideration of winegrowers' needs by equipment designers.

The combination of epidemiology and ergotoxicology has made it possible to better characterize pesticide contamination by focusing on real work situations, where multiple exposures intertwine (Garrigou et al. 2011). The surface area treated (number of hectares), which is generally one of the variables used in epidemiology to measure the degree of exposure, has been supplemented by the inclusion of ergonomic criteria in the characterization and measurement of pesticide exposure (Garrigou et al. 2008).

This approach enabled us to identify variations in contamination depending on the individual and the work situation, and to objectify the variation in exposure from one work organization to another. Professional expertise, whether it be individual or collective, developed and capitalized on during the course of experience (Garrigou 2011), can be seen as a determining factor in situations of exposure or non-exposure. These also include contaminations linked to people's natural habits (scratching their face, touching their mouth, onychophagy, etc.), linked to a preconceived idea of how to avoid exposure. We were also able to identify and explain contamination related to equipment design faults (positioning of controls, seals, nozzle clogging, etc.) or to a lack of advice on the use, maintenance and cleaning of PPE. This kind of work practice characterization has been used to inform prevention programs in winegrowing environments (Garrigou et al. 2005, 2006).

1.3.2. *Ergotoxicology's contribution to understanding situations involving pesticide risk*

1.3.2.1. *The ARC-CMR agricultural project*

An analysis of the social construction of workplace prevention of carcinogenic, mutagenic and reprotoxic (CMR) risk was carried out as part of the ARC-CMR project. This project, funded by the Association pour la recherche sur le cancer (ARC)[2] between 2013 and 2016, was carried out by ergotoxicologists from the EPICENE-INSERM team in Bordeaux, in collaboration with the Agence nationale d'amélioration des conditions de travail (ANACT)[3] and the Agences régionales (ARACT) Aquitaine, Corse et Picardie[4]. In this example, we focus on the results

2 Cancer Research Association.

3 French National Agency for the Improvement of Working Conditions.

4 Regional agencies (ARACT) in Aquitaine, Corsica and Picardy.

produced in the agricultural environment with regard to chlorpropham (CIPC), a pesticide used in the cultivation and preservation of potatoes.

The ARC-CMR project presents CMR risk prevention levers based on an analysis of real work by farmers. Observation of work situations supported the documentation of CMR risk representations. It also enabled us to discuss the influence of the system of actors surrounding farms on the prevention of a vague, diffuse and indirect risk. These two objects of study were linked to the farmers' actual activities, in order to understand how this social construction of CMR risks could promote or hinder prevention in real work situations.

The ergotoxicological approach was used by the ARC-CMR project to highlight exposure under real conditions of the use of plant protection products. The results of the targeted metrology were used to discuss the determinants of pesticide exposure with the farmers observed, and their spouses. Here, we present the construction of the metrology in potato thermonebulization (or thermal fogging), so as to reveal and discuss situations of pesticide risk with farmers and those around them. We base our argument on unpublished research reports by Galey et al. (2015) and Théry et al. (2015).

1.3.2.2. *Thermonebulization*

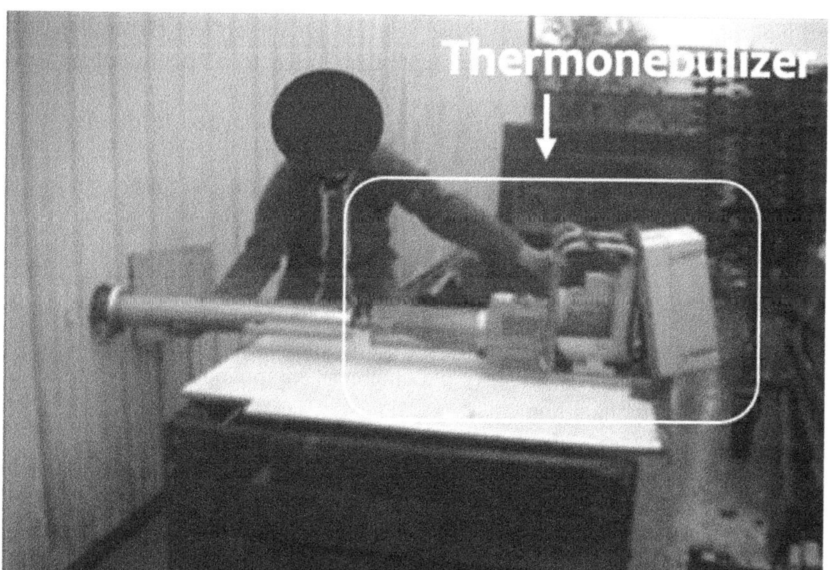

Figure 1.4. *Thermal fogger inserted into the wall of the potato storage building. Observation of January 16, 2014, farm B. For a color version of this figure, see www.iste.co.uk/botero/pesticides.zip*

Thermal fogging is used to protect potatoes from sprouting. It involves "gassing" potatoes that have been harvested and then stored at low temperature in a building. Harvests stored from November to May are mainly destined for industrial use. Depending on the product used and the desired storage time, the potatoes are gassed 2–10 times a year during the winter and spring.

The device used is a thermal fogger (Figure 1.4). The device works by passing an anti-sprouting product in a liquid state over a hot resistor, vaporizing the liquid and allowing an aerosol of fine droplets to settle around the potatoes to be treated. The mist of droplets, a few microns in diameter, needs to be diffused into the storage area through the building's internal ventilation. Weather conditions with little wind are favorable. In fact, the success of the operation depends on the air tightness of the treated building, and the proper distribution and circulation of steam within it. Strong winds can disrupt the air flow and lead to vapor losses outside the storage building.

1.3.2.3. *Ergotoxicology approach*

1.3.2.3.1. Work observations combined with metrology

Observations took place during three thermal fogging sessions between January and February 2014. Two of these took place on the same farm (farm plot A). The third took place on a farm outside those selected for the project (farm plot B). The aim of this third observation was to compare practices and identify variability.

We present here the targeted metrology protocol designed to observe thermal fogging activity combined with metrology.

Before each observation, the ergotoxicologist's workflow was presented to the professional being monitored. Each person under observation was fitted with a heart rate monitor at the start of the operation. This was followed by an initial "white" handwash before the professional began to touch their equipment (in other words, before the equipment was removed from storage or the premises opened). The purpose of this wash was to identify the chemical compounds that were present on the hands prior to any handling.

Subsequent handwashes enabled us to identify the elements that were present on the hands during handling, and to observe any variations. The second and third handwashes were carried out after installation and removal of the thermal fogger. The last wash took place at the very end of the activity.

The camera starts recording from the first handwash until the end of the treatment activity. The participants then film the activities of the professional farmers. The shots and actions filmed correspond to previously established hypotheses. These are situations in which professionals have to refill the thermal fogger (three- to five five-liter cans are put into the device for one treatment). The assembly and disassembly phases of the thermal fogger are also filmed, as they involve skin contact.

Agreement to use fluorescein was obtained for all observations. Three fluorescein granules (for a volume of 25 liters of product) were mixed with a bottle of mineral water (50 cl) to dissolve the granules. The mixture was then added to the first can of plant protection product used that day by the professional.

As soon as all of the canisters had been used, an initial test with the UV lamp was carried out (in the dark). The lamp was passed over the upper part of the body, coveralls and shoes of the professional being monitored. A second test was carried out once the equipment had been dismantled and put away.

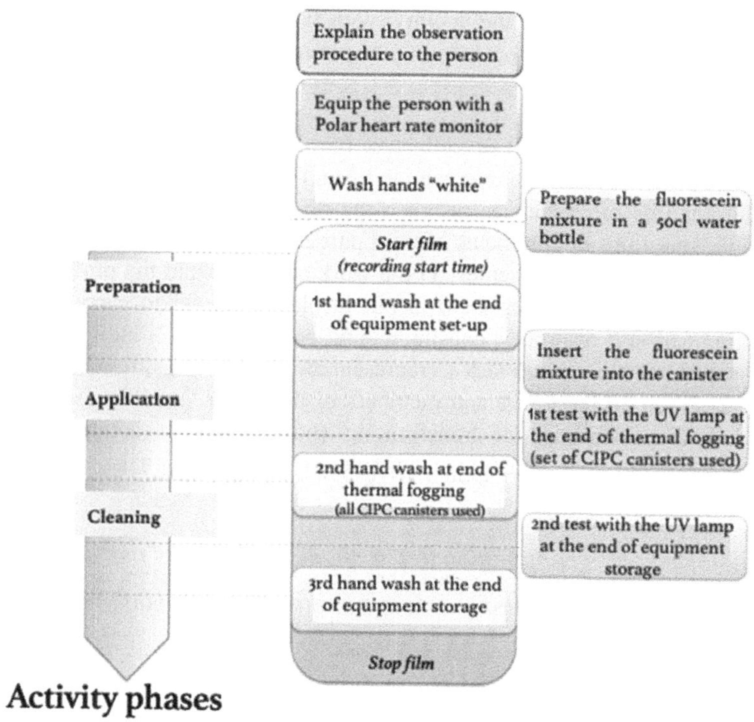

Figure 1.5. *Representation of the application of metrology tools used for the analysis of thermal fogger activity (2015). For a color version of this figure, see www.iste.co.uk/botero/pesticides.zip*

Figure 1.5 shows a schematic of the targeted metrology carried out for the thermal fogger activity on each of the farms.

1.3.2.3.2. Individual interviews and group discussions based on the results of targeted metrology

Self-confrontation interviews and exchanges between professionals and those around them were proposed to each of the farmers. The discussions were based on a variety of aids, designed to help them recall or contextualize their work situations (video montages, measurement results, field notes, safety data sheets, etc.). The individual interviews ended with a discussion on perceived risks and a shared reflection on the crop protection product used on the day of the filmed observation. Following these interviews, and after validation by the professionals observed in the images in the montage, the discussion based on the results of the targeted metrology was proposed to other actors, both internal and external to the farm (other farmers carrying out the treatment activity and their spouses). Observation materials were discussed with external actors of the activity, with the aim of building prevention and developing shared reflection on potential or proven risk situations, beyond the time of the intervention.

Whether individual (one hour) or collective (two to three hours), the sessions were filmed and transcribed by the intervention team. Post-viewing and transcription supported the analysis of exchanges between the professional, the image of their activity, and the questions or comments of third parties. The analysis based on these materials was built around four themes: 1) the work activity (what the professional puts in place and what it requires them to put in place in order to carry out the thermal fogging activity: resources, constraints and possibilities); 2) individual and collective exposure to pesticides (representations, feelings, experiences, interviewing both the professionals and members of the farm); 3) self-preservation strategies; and 4) possibilities of transforming (possibilities of action on the determinants) pesticide risk situations encountered by professionals and those around them.

1.3.2.4. *Ergotoxicology's contribution to the characterization of risk situations*

1.3.2.4.1. Regulations concerning chlorpropham (CIPC) used in thermal fogging operations

In each case, chlorpropham-based phytopharmaceutical products (CIPC) were used as anti-germinants to treat the 1,000 tons of stored potatoes. Commercial products used to thermally fog potatoes meet the definition of a plant protection product, as stipulated in Regulation (EC) No. 1107/2009 concerning the placing of plant protection products on the market. After an initial European review, CIPC was approved as a sprout inhibitor on February 1, 2005. In 2019, it was withdrawn from the market following findings by the European Food Safety Authority (EFSA) of potentially harmful exposure to this substance and one of its metabolites, 3-chloroaniline, and uncertainty about possible endocrine-disrupting properties.

During our observations in 2014, CIPC was classified as R40 and a category 2 carcinogen according to the European classification, with risks of serious health effects in the event of prolonged exposure by ingestion. The safety data sheets indicated that the routes of exposure were by inhalation and skin contact. Recommended protective measures included good ventilation of the building being treated, wearing appropriate gloves, protective clothing and safety glasses, and the use of a respiratory device in the event of inadequate ventilation of the premises.

Additional information found on the manufacturer's website specifies that the aerosols generated consist of droplets of 0.1–5 μm. This aerosol particle size is of particular concern because of the possibility of it being deposited in the pulmonary alveoli.

1.3.2.4.2. Characterization of pesticide exposure using fluorescein tests and handwashing

Fluorescein tests did not reveal any skin exposure. Yellow fluorescent highlights were only detected in one of the three cases (thermal fogging operation B).

The analytical results of the handwashed water samples taken were below the detection thresholds for the tests performed. A long delay between sample collection and laboratory analysis may also explain the results obtained (e.g. the degradation of chlorpropham). Another possibility is that handwashing at too high a frequency may not detect the presence and exposure of the substance at the microgram level. Under these conditions, it is not possible to draw any quantitative conclusions about exposure in relation to the activity performed.

In the laboratory, handwashed water was tested for additional active ingredients. Traces of 22 substances used in the composition of pesticides were present in the farmers' handwashed water. Concentrations were in the μg/l range. Although these values are well below the AOEL (Acceptable Operator Exposure Level), questions arise regarding the age of the sample: samples were taken more than six months after the last field spraying. Identifying the origin of these exposures is complex. Further investigations need to be carried out to pinpoint their possible origins.

Current data on chlorpropham and technological advances suggest that we should replicate this approach in the future, looking for the chlorpropham metabolite (3-chloroaniline), supplementing handwashing with surface sampling and requesting laboratory analysis at sub-microgram levels for a whole range of pesticides.

1.3.2.4.3. Understanding exposure through analysis of cardiac costs during activity

Significant cardiac costs were noted in all observations of thermal fogging activity, particularly in the equipment setup and storage phases. The cardiac cost measured corresponds to a heavy to very heavy level, with a score of 14 and 15 corresponding to the maximum level of the Meunier grid (Meunier et al. 1994).

These costs can be explained by the configuration of the installations. On farm A (observations 1 and 2), the thermal fogger was placed high up on a walkway. Installation was carried out manually by the farmer, requiring them to carry the thermal fogger upstairs or on a ladder. A heart rate level higher than 80% (152 bpm) of the theoretical maximum heart rate was recorded (Figure 1.6).

The values presented could only be increased under optimum protection conditions, where the operator would be equipped with a suit and mask. The use of a respirator with physical intensity levels, such as those found on farm site A, would lead to leakage of the seal, minimizing protection. The use of coveralls would increase physical strain, leading to higher heart and respiratory rates.

The variations recorded between the situations observed can be explained by individual characteristics such as different sporting practices, as well as by the strategies and expertise developed by people in the activity, for example, in carrying the thermal fogger.

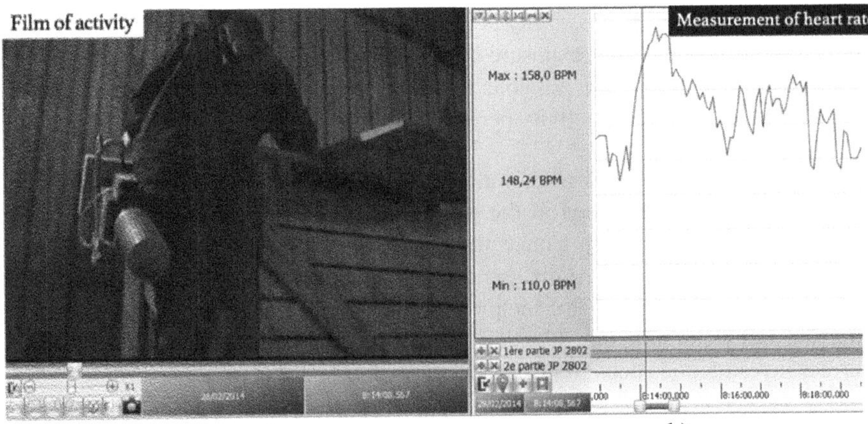

a) b)

Figure 1.6. *Video of activity synchronized with heart rate measurement. a) Installation of thermal fogger, b) heart rate reading at 152 bpm, February 28, 2014, farm B. For a color version of this figure, see www.iste.co.uk/botero/pesticides.zip*

1.3.2.4.4. Analysis of pesticide risk situations based on the film of the activity discussed with the monitored farmers

Skin contact with CIPC was observed on the thermal fogger, the glass wool used to caulk the premises, the used canisters, the knife and cutter used to pierce the products, the table supporting the thermal fogger, the work clothes and the box used to transport the device in the professional's vehicle.

Figures 1.7–1.9 show these contacts between working people and soiled surfaces.

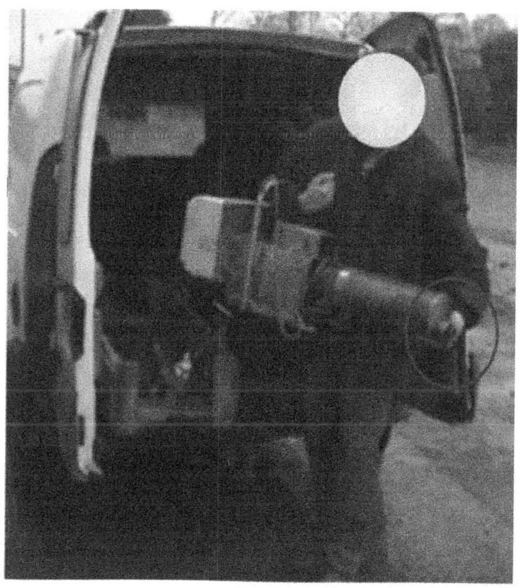

Figure 1.7. *Unloading the thermal fogger. Hand contact with barrel. 11:50 a.m., January 15, 2014, farm A. For a color version of this figure, see www.iste.co.uk/botero/pesticides.zip*

After unloading and installing the thermal fogger on the walkway adjoining the building where the potatoes are stored, the farmer went to the other side of the wall to check their equipment, particularly that the end of the cannon was positioned correctly. They explained that the expected gaseous form of CIPC remains liquid until the device is "hot enough". We then watched them install a CIPC drip tray (Figure 1.8) and come into contact with the pre-treated potatoes. In January 2020, EFSA published a report stating that, in the case of chlorpropham, in warehouses where potatoes have been stored and treated for many years, the walls and floors contain residues of this substance, which can be released. As of yet, no cleaning protocol has been found that has proved capable of rendering warehouses totally residue-free. It is therefore likely that the traces of pesticide found on the farmer's hands during the thermal fogging operation may have come from contact with previously treated potatoes. For example, when potatoes are grown, before they are harvested, they are topkilled using a product generally classified as CMR category 2. Thus, during potato sorting and storage, potential exposure could occur through residual dusts that are potentially contaminated by the products used before and after harvesting.

CIPC emissions outside buildings are a real problem for the farmers we met (Figure 1.9). In fact, exposure resulting from leaking premises was observed on all three of the thermal fogging locations monitored. The use of glass wool to reinforce waterproofing reduces exposure to CIPC vapors. However, by installing and removing the glass wool, the farmer is indirectly exposed to CIPC by handling the glass wool with their bare hands. Furthermore, the effectiveness of the glass wool does not appear to be sufficient, due to the fog observed in the farmer's untreated shed (farm A). A strong odor was present throughout the treatment period and remained for several weeks after our observations.

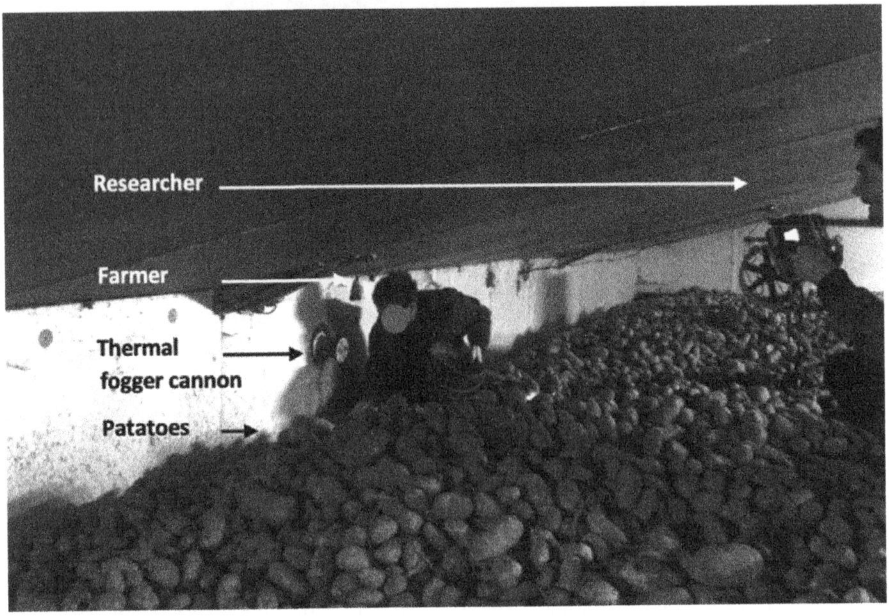

Figure 1.8. *Installation of a CIPC retention bucket under the cannon prior to thermally fogging potatoes, January 15, 2014, farm A. For a color version of this figure, see www.iste.co.uk/botero/pesticides.zip*

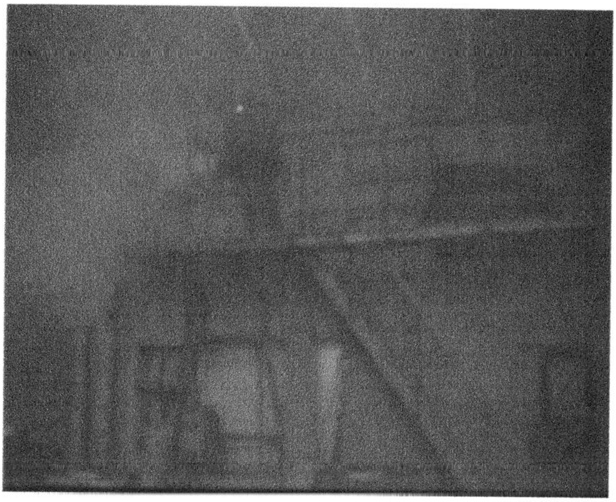

Figure 1.9. *Unexpected release of CIPC fog around the farmer, on the other side of the building where potatoes are processed. 10:32 a.m., January 15, 2014, farm A. For a color version of this figure, see www.iste.co.uk/botero/pesticides.zip*

To unclog the thermal fogger and clean the plant protection product sampling tube, farmer A went home during the activity. They needed water to restart the device. In this situation, the question of contamination of the farmer's private sphere was particularly relevant. The filming of the activity showed the body as a vehicle (Mohammed-Brahim 2009), in which the deposited substance can be transmitted from one part of the body to another, as well as to distant spaces such as the domestic environment. The question of indirect contact with elements of the farmer's private sphere also arose during discussions with the farmers observed. Indeed, proximity to the home can lead to migration of active matter to one of the transfers of contamination (contact with the handle, computer and desk, coffee machine, vehicle, knife, etc.). Work clothes being washed at home also raise questions for all farming operations.

Observations of direct and indirect contact with the product are confirmed by the farmers. All direct and related handling operations of the thermal fogger are recorded. Oily contact with the barrel of the thermal fogger is well highlighted in the activity descriptions. In order to work on the equipment, farmers entering the building where the active thermal fogger is located move through clouds of CIPC. These inhalation exposures mainly occur during the refueling phases of the thermal fogger. The need to refill, as well as the risk of fire associated with the equipment's temperature rise (350°C), prompt the farmers observed to stay close to their equipment.

For the farmers we met, thermal fogging remains an occasional activity, for which safety and prevention practices built on repeated treatments are not observed. The advice given by both the plant protection product manufacturer and the farmers' mutual insurance company is only partially applied, as it is complex to implement during the activity (cleaning the gun after each use, carrying out the operation by a specialized service provider, etc.).

1.3.2.4.5. Discussing the determinants of pesticide exposure with farmers

Three main ways of representing pesticide risk seem to be emerging. The first is primarily represented by the senses, by bodily experience of the product; a product that we can see or smell, or whose short-term effects we have experienced, making the risk "palpable". The second way is through cognitive construction, through empirical or statistical evidence of health effects. The fact that little is known about the real effects of CIPC and the lack of formal data in 2014 may have been a major obstacle to risk prevention. The final avenue is discussion forums, which appear to be the most effective channel for risk awareness.

During the interviews, farmers spoke of the importance of having discussion forums where they could not only discuss the subject of CMRs, but also debate and share experiences. "It's a place for exchange, and that counts for a lot". For the farmers we interviewed, the subject of chemical risk is still rarely brought up spontaneously in informal circles (acquaintances, family), hence the importance of relying on structured discussion forums (led, for example, by associations or possibly players in the prevention network). The results of the metrology study, coupled with the video footage of the activity, enabled them to verify their findings on exposure, to remove some of the vagueness surrounding CMR exposure, and to work together to identify actions to be taken to reduce risks.

Ergotoxicology helped farmers to take a step back from their activities and the associated risks. The approach enabled them to observe that, even at stages of production when they thought they had the risk under control, conventional and regulated prevention measures were not sufficient to protect themselves properly, and even led to cross-contamination through protective equipment. Measurements and discussions with farmers, and those around them, have enabled us to identify areas for improvement in relation to the actual work and day-to-day life of the people involved (e.g. separation of professional and personal areas, or use of clothing dedicated to treatments).

Based on the activity films produced, the determinants of treatment activity were discussed with the farmers and those around them, and actions to be taken beyond the farm level were devised to take preventive action. For example, it was decided to renegotiate the specifications imposed by industrial buyers of potatoes, and to seek solutions to ensure that the thermal fogging activity was no longer outsourced to farmers. There has also been talk of mobilizing manufacturers of agricultural machinery and phytopharmaceutical products: to improve label reading by highlighting information on risks; to improve the usability of packaging, particularly in terms of weight, grip and opening system, in order to limit the risks of splashing and spillage; to incorporate a colorant and an odorant additive into products, enabling toxicity to be perceived during use, etc.

In addition, machine manufacturers have a role to play in improving the organization of the farmers' work, through technical developments that optimize hygiene and organization during the use of their equipment, such as the introduction of systems which allow farmers to avoid having to refill with plant protection products during treatments.

1.3.2.5. *Summary*

With the first example, we were able to observe how the coupling of pesticide metrology with the analysis of work situations was able to challenge conventional pesticide risk assessment methods. The results of this pairing were used to mobilize various pesticide prevention bodies (Garrigou 2011), as well as to open up preventative action beyond simple training in good practices for chemical product users. The traces of the activity, built up in a multi-disciplinary way, have thus provided a group of researchers with solid arguments for creating a formidable awareness process with regard to the reliability of protective equipment and the assessment of exposure under real conditions of use.

The second example shows how targeted metrology can help farmers to become more autonomous in identifying situations involving risk. Revealing traces of pesticide residues and contact between people (during and outside the activity) gives substance to exposure. The tools of ergotoxicology are an asset to prevention, as they help represent risks. The self-confrontation interview also revealed the conditions under which exposure situations are produced, and encouraged collective discussion of the work, its reality and its constraints, with a view to taking preventive action and empowering working people.

1.4. Contributions and limits of ergotoxicology to the characterization of pesticide exposure

> The organizations responsible for assessing and controlling risks are structurally dependent on scientific disciplines and instruments guiding the way they see – and fail to see – the dangers they must prevent (Dedieu and Jouzel 2015, p. 106).

Hazards are reduced to their most easily quantifiable dimensions, and available but poorly compatible knowledge "is excluded from the control systems on which public authorities rely to identify and prevent health risks" (Dedieu and Jouzel 2015, p. 106). However, in a context where several factors will interact, a crucial issue in exposure assessment is also to provide information on the context, tasks or exposing activities (Sznelwar 1992; Mohammed-Brahim 1996; Garrigou et al. 2008).

The toxicological models used to estimate exposure values provide a framework for tackling occupational health problems caused by the use of plant protection products and cannot themselves guarantee the safety of their users. By incorporating "a highly prescriptive vision of tasks involving contact with pesticides", these models perpetuate "a vision according to which poor practices of agricultural workers are the causes of poisoning – and not the products" (LISIS 2017).

The marketing authorization (MA) system for plant protection products, and the models on which it is based, have limitations and weaknesses that have serious consequences for prevention. We note a significant gap between the situations modeled during this "upstream" assessment and the reality of situations of use documented by the ergotoxicological approach. This gap raises questions about the diversity of sociotechnical and cultural contexts of real-life situations, and how these are considered in the situations modeled.

The activity concept should involve matching the needs and capabilities of those undertaking the work with the tasks they are expected to perform (Goutille et al. 2024). This chapter has provided an in-depth examination of the impact of this unsuitability on the incidence of pesticide exposure in plant protection product use. In the two examples presented, the actual conditions of pesticide exposure call into question the classic organization and management logics of pesticide risk, prompting us to invest work activity beyond the scope of the company.

Ergotoxicology, in its developmental aim, seeks to help people in the workplace to understand the harmfulness of their working environment and to transform it, based on their concerns and pre-occupation (Goutille 2022). With its approach and tools focused on real work activity, ergotoxicology produces sufficiently specific data to induce preventive action, at the level of work and life situations and with the system of actors who prescribe the farmers' work (Jolly and Goutille 2024). The subjective commitment of researchers and farmers is called upon to take charge of what the administrative and territorial organization cannot resolve on the initial issue of exposure. In fact, ergotoxicology cannot do without multidisciplinary collaboration to "instrument action on the production process itself" (Sznelwar 1992), nor can it do without transprofessional collaborations with farmers to take preventive action, here and now.

1.5. References

Albert, M. (2018). Une approche critique de la conception et des usages du matériel de pulvérisation des pesticides en viticulture. Apport de l'approche instrumentale à l'ergotoxicologie pour la conception. Ergonomics Master's Thesis, Conservatoire national des arts et métiers, Bordeaux.

Baldi, I., Lebailly, P., Rondeau, V., Bouchart, V., Blanc-Lapierre, A., Bouvier, G., Canal-Raffin, M., Garrigou, A. (2012). Levels and determinants of pesticide exposure in operators involved in treatment of vineyards: Results of the PESTEXPO study. *Journal of Exposure Analysis and Environmental Epidemiology*, 22(6), 593–600.

Baldi, I., Lebailly, P., Bouvier, G., Rondeau, V., Kientz-Bouchart, V., Canal-Raffin, M., Garrigou, A. (2014). Levels and determinants of pesticide exposure in re-entry workers in vineyards: Results of the PESTEXPO study. *Environmental Research*, 132, 360–369.

Baldi, I., Berthet, A., Garrigou, A., Jas, N., Jouzel, J-N., Lebailly, P., Martin, A., Moquay, V., Prete, G., Tudori, L. (2023). Pour une expertise scientifique et technique impartiale en vue de la maîtrise des expositions professionnelles aux pesticides en milieu agricole. Final Report of the specific formation of Commission nationale de la déontologie et des alertes en matière de santé publique et d'environnement (cnDAspe).

Baratta, R. (1997). Filmer le travail : de quel travail s'agit-il ? *Champs Visuels*, 6, 94–110.

Béguin, P. (1997). Le caméscope, l'image et le mot. Quelques remarques sur l'usage de la vidéo pour l'analyse du travail. *Champs Visuels*, 6, 60–68.

Béguin, P. (2004). Mondes, monde commun et versions des mondes. *Bulletin de psychologie*, 57(469), 45–48.

Brown, O. (2005). Participatory ergonomics. In *Handbook of Human Factors and Ergonomics Methods*, Stanton, N. et al. (eds). CRC Press, Boca Raton.

Callon, M., Lascoumes, P., Barthe, Y. (2001). *Agir dans un monde incertain. Essai sur la démocratie technique*. Le Seuil, Paris.

Clot, Y. (1999). *La fonction psychologique du travail*. PUF, Paris.

Clot, Y. and Granger, B. (2019). Restaurer l'initiative collective au service de la santé psychique. *Psychiatrie Sciences Humaines Neurosciences*, 17(1), 15–32.

Daniellou, F. (1997). Évolutions de l'ergonomie francophone : théories, pratiques et théories de la pratique. *Actes du 32ème Congrès de la SELF*, 37–54.

Dedieu, F. and Jouzel, J.-N. (2015). Comment ignorer ce que l'on sait : la domestication des savoirs inconfortables sur les intoxications des agriculteurs par les pesticides. *Revue française de sociologie*, 56(1), 105–133.

Duraffourg, J. and Vuillon, B. (2004). *Alain Wisner et les tâches du présent. La bataille du travail réel*. Octarès Éditions, Toulouse.

Falzon, P. (2004). Nature, objectifs et connaissances de l'ergonomie. In *Ergonomie*, Falzon, P. (ed.). PUF, Paris, 15–35.

French Ministry of Agriculture (2006). Analyse et synthèse des contrôles réalisés en 2003 et 2004 concernant le respect de la réglementation de protection de la santé, lors de l'utilisation des produits phytosanitaires au sein des entreprises agricoles. Note DGFAR/SDTE/N2006-5029.

Fucks, I. and Bourmaud, L. (2011). L'écran, l'alarme et la culture. *Actes du 46ème Congrès de la SELF*, 201–206.

Galey, L., Goutille, F., Rambaud, C. (2015). Rapport de terrains agricoles de l'équipe transversale. Projet ANACT 2014-2016. Unpublished.

Galey, L., Judon, N., Jolly, C., Goutille, F., Morelot, S., Albert, M., Lhospital, O., Martin, P., Noel-Suberville, C., Pasquereau, P. et al. (2019). Proposition méthodologique en ergotoxicologie pour révéler les expositions à des produits chimiques. *Activités*, 16(1). doi: 10.4000/activites.4103.

Galey, L., Audignon, S., Witschger, O., Bau, S., Judon, N., Lacourt, A., Garrigou, A. (2020). What does ergonomics have to do with nanotechnologies? A case study. *Applied Ergonomics*, 87(103116). doi: 10.1016/j.apergo.2020.103116.

Garrigou, A. (2011). Le développement de l'ergotoxicologie. Une contribution de l'ergonomie à la santé au travail. HDR Thesis, Université de Bordeaux, Bordeaux.

Garrigou, A., Mohammed-Brahim, B., Daniellou, F. (1998). Étude ergonomique sur les chantiers de déflocage d'amiante. Final Report, OPPBTP/DRT.CT3, Bordeaux.

Garrigou, A., Baldi, I., Satoura, C., Rougetet, L., Nicolay, A., Duverneix, C. (2005). Élaboration d'un processus de formation aux risques liés à l'usage des produits phytosanitaires dans la viticulture. *Actes du 40ème Congrès de la SELF*.

Garrigou, A., Baldi, I., Rougetet, L. (2006). Developing a training module against the risks associated with the use of phytosanitary substances in the wine-growing industry. In *Meeting Diversity in Ergnonomics*, Pikaar, R.N., Koningsveld, E., Settels, P. (eds). Elsevier, Amsterdam.

Garrigou, A., Baldi, I., Dubuc, P. (2008). Apports de l'ergotoxicologie à l'évaluation de l'efficacité réelle des EPI devant protéger du risque phytosanitaire : de l'analyse de la contamination au processus collectif d'alerte. *Perspectives interdisciplinaires sur le travail et la santé*, 10(1). doi: 10.4000/pistes.2137.

Garrigou, A., Baldi, I., Le Frious, P., Anselm, R., Vallier, M. (2011). Ergonomics contribution to chemical risks prevention: An ergotoxicological investigation of the effectiveness of coverall against plant pest risk in viticulture. *Applied Ergonomics*. 42(2), 321–330. doi: 10.1016/j.apergo.2010.08.001.

Garrigou, A., Théry, L., Chassaing, K., Effantin, E., Mercieca, P., Dimerman, S., Vanderghote, M., Négroni, P., Gauthier, P., Goutille, F. et al. (2015). Une approche pluridisciplinaire du processus de construction sociale de la prévention du risque CMR. *Actes du 50ème Congrès de la SELF*, 476–489.

Garrigou, A., Judon, N., Goutille, F., Galey, L., Gruénais, M.-E., Mohammed Brahim, B., Jackson, M. (2017). Les représentations des risques comme objet de dialogue pour construire la prévention. *52ème Congrès de la SELF.*

Gatignol, C. and Étienne, J.-C. (2010). Pesticides et santé. Report, Office parlementaire d'évaluation des choix scientifiques et technologiques.

Goutille, F. (2022). Ne plus ignorer les agriculteurs : une contribution de l'ergonomie à la prévention du risque pesticides en milieu viticole. PhD Thesis, Université de Bordeaux, Bordeaux.

Goutille, F. and Garrigou, A. (2021). Traitements phytosanitaires en viticulture française et prévention du risque pesticides. Retour d'expérience d'une communauté élargie de recherche ayant mobilisé l'ergotoxicologie. *VertigO – la revue électronique en sciences de l'environnement*, 21(3).

Goutille, F., Galey, L., Rambaud, C., Pasquereau, P., Filho J.M.J., Garrigou, A. (2016). Prescrição e utilização de equipamentos de proteção individual (EPI) em atividades com exposição a produtos químicos cancerígenos, mutagênicos e reprotóxicos (CMR): pesquisa-ação pluridisciplinar em uma fábrica francesa de decoração para móveis. Os equipamentos de proteção individual (EPI): protetores, mas nem sempre. *Laboreal*, 12(1), 23–38.

Goutille, F., Degbelo, A.N., Calleja, C., Garrigou, A., Candau, J. (2024). Online collaborative research on seasonal work. Collective capabilities to resist on precarious work and living conditions. *Work*. doi: 10.3233/WOR-230744.

Guérin, F., Pueyo, V., Béguin, P., Garrigou, A., Hubault, F., Maline, J., Morlet, T. (2021). *Concevoir le travail, le défi de l'ergonomie.* Éditions Octarès, Toulouse.

Jolly, C. (2022). Les pratiques professionnelles des propriétaires exploitants agricoles, ressources pour limiter l'exposition cutanée aux pesticides ? PhD Thesis, Université du Québec à Montréal.

Jolly, C. and Goutille, F. (2024). Comparaison de l'activité de travail d'agriculteurs québécois et français pour comprendre l'exposition aux pesticides. In *Exposition aux pesticides. Ce qu'en disent les sciences humaines et sociales*, Goutille, F., Lambert, E., Candau, J. (eds). Octares Éditions, Toulouse.

Jouzel, J.-N. (2019). *Pesticides. Comment ignorer ce que l'on sait.* Presses de Sciences Po, Paris.

Jouzel, J.-N. and Dedieu, F. (2011). L'ergotoxicologie est-elle soluble dans les politiques de prévention du risque chimique professionnel ? Le cas de l'"enquête arsénite de soude" et de ses (in)-conséquences réglementaires. *Actes du 46ème Congrès de la SELF*, 254–260.

Judon, N. (2017). Rendre possible un espace intermédiaire de dialogue pour co construire de nouvelles solutions de prévention dans un contexte d'incertitude. Cas des travaux de revêtements routiers. PhD Thesis, Université de Bordeaux, Bordeaux.

Laurent, C., Baldi, I., Bernadac, G., Berthet, A., Colosio, C., Garrigou, A., Grimbuhler, S., Guichard, L., Jas, N., Jouzel, J.-N. et al. (2016). Expositions professionnelles aux pesticides en agriculture. Collective Expertise Report, Agence nationale de sécurité sanitaire de l'alimentation, de l'environnement et du travail.

Le Bossé, Y. (2012). *Sortir de l'impuissance : invitation à soutenir le développement du pouvoir d'agir des personnes et des collectivités. Tome 1 : fondements et cadres conceptuels*. Ardis Publishing, New York.

Lebailly, P., Bouchart, V., Baldi, I., Lecluse, Y., Heutte, N., Gislard, A., Malas, J.-P. (2009). Exposure to pesticides in open-field farming in France. *Annals of Occupational Hygiene*, 53(1), 69–81.

LISIS (2017). Usage des modèles dans l'évaluation des risques des produits chimiques. Report, INRS.

Meunier, P., Smolik, H.J., Knoche, C. (1994). Astreinte cardiaque et travail. Quelle grille d'évaluation choisir ? *Cahiers de médecine interprofessionnelle*, 34(2), 153–158.

Mohammed-Brahim, B. (1996). Du point de vue du travail ou comment sulfater la vigne autrement : approche ergotoxicologique du traitement phytosanitaire en viticulture. Master's Thesis in Ergonomics, Université de Bordeaux 2, Bordeaux.

Mohammed-Brahim, B. (2000). Concept and methods in ergotoxicology. *International Encyclopedia of Ergonomics and Human Factors*, 1, 698–705.

Mohammed-Brahim, B. (2004). Ergotoxicologie : de la connaissance à l'action. *Journées annuelles de la société de médecine du travail de Midi-Pyrénées*, Toulouse.

Mohammed-Brahim, B. (2006). Étude ergotoxicologique de l'exposition aux mycotoxines lors des opérations de broyage des graines préalablement à leur analyse. Study Report, CETAPP.

Mohammed-Brahim, B. (2009). Travailler en présence de substances toxiques : un corps à corps au quotidien. *Corps au travail*, 6(1), 53–59.

Mohammed-Brahim, B. and Garrigou, A. (2009). Une approche critique du modèle dominant de prévention du risque chimique : l'apport de l'ergotoxicologie. *Activités*, 6(1). doi: 10.4000/activites.2086.

Nascimento, A., Cuvelier, L., Mollo, V., Dicciocio, A., Falzon, P. (2013). Constructing safety: From the normative to the adaptive view. In *Constructive Ergonomics*, Falzon, P. (ed.). CRC Press, Taylor & Francis Group, Boca Raton.

OECD (1997). *Guidance Document for the Conduct of Studies of Occupational Exposure to Pesticides During Agricultural Application*. OECD, Paris.

Sznelwar, L.I. (1992). Analyse ergonomique de l'exposition de travailleurs agricoles aux pesticides : essai ergotoxicologique. Ergonomics PhD Thesis, CNAM de Paris, Paris.

Théry, L., Effantin, E., Vanderghote, M., Mercieca, P., Baratta, R., Galey, L., Goutille, F., Rambaud, C. (2015). Une approche pluridisciplinaire du processus de construction sociale du risque CMR. *Actes du 50ème Congrès de la SELF*.

Theureau, J. (2010). Les entretiens d'autoconfrontation et de remise en situation par les traces matérielles et le programme de recherche "cours d'action". *Revue d'anthropologie des connaissances*, 4(2), 287–322.

Van Belleghem, L. (2015). La convocation de l'activité : une méthode d'analyse au service de la discussion. *Le travail humain*, 79(3), 285–306.

Vézina, N. (2001). La pratique de l'ergonomie face aux TMS : ouverture à l'interdisciplinarité. *Comptes rendus du congrès SELF-ACE 2001 – Les transformations du travail, enjeux pour l'ergonomie*, 44–60.

Villatte, R. (1983). Pour une ergo-toxicologie. *19ème Congrès de la SELF.*

Vink, P., Koningsveld, E.A.P., Molenbroek, J.F. (2006). Positive outcomes of participatory ergonomics in terms of greater comfort and higher productivity. *Applied Ergonomics*, 37, 537–546.

2

Thinking about Pesticides in Terms of a "Socio-technical Lock-in" of Information

2.1. Introduction

Following on from the Grenelle de l'environnement (2007) and the related programming law of August 3, 2009, the Écophyto 2018 plan (2009–2015) aimed to reduce the use of plant protection products in agriculture by 50% by 2018. In a report from November 17, 2019, the Cour des Comptes points out that the targets for reducing the use of plant protection products set out in the Écophyto 2018 plan (and its subsequent versions Écophyto II and Écophyto II+) are a long way from being achieved[1], and specifies that the initial target has been postponed until 2025[2]. These disappointing results raise questions about the reasons for this failure, and inspire proposals for ways forward. The NA'Stras and Phyt'Info projects led by the University of Strasbourg[3] are in line with these proposals, in particular those aimed at improving knowledge and tools for tomorrow, and supporting the information provided to consumers on the sanitary quality of food products. The aim of these projects is to examine how digital information formats on plant protection products can help us to promote more sustainable practices. The work presented here focuses more specifically on digital food guidance devices for consumers. In a first exploratory phase, we carried out a census and review of these devices to inventory the way in which sites and applications take hold of elements for qualifying the quality of food products. In addition to this documentary analysis, we conducted qualitative interviews with digital device owners. The categorization exercise, such as the associated

Chapter written by Jan SMOLINSKI.

1 See: www.ccomptes.fr/fr/publications/le-bilan-des-plans-ecophyto.

2 A project on alternatives to plant protection products launched in May 2023 should contribute to the construction of the Ecophyto 2030 plan.

3 See: https://numali.unistra.fr.

analysis, and the interview support show that in the message designed to show a "good product", communication related to the use/nonuse of pesticides is discrete, appearing to be exposed to an informational lock-in (Callon and Ferrary 2006), a barrier that must no doubt be correlated to a fear of foodstuffs being disqualified under tense markets (Geiger et al. 2014). As a counterpoint to this observation, we have turned our attention to players who, contrary to these tensions, have sought ways of circumventing this obstacle. Expectations of healthy food, which integrates the preservation of ecosystems, come up against the need for accessible and reliable information. Questioning the design of communication aimed at consumers therefore leads us to consider, in the context of claims on pesticides and more generally on food quality, the preservation (versus waste) of consumers' cognitive and organizational resources, and the desired effects on decision-making processes.

2.2. Communicating using the term *pesticide*: why and how?

Why and how can we communicate with consumers while mentioning the term pesticide as part of a socio-technical labeling[4] (Laurent and Mallard 2020)? In a context where the attempt to constitute "a narrative relating to the protection of plants and the prosperity of the human species [...] is now undermined by the health and ecological consequences of pesticides" (Botero 2021, p. 104), the NA'Stras and Phyt'Info[5] projects aim to shed light on the subject by questioning the ways in which

4 The term *labeling* here is understood as referring to a process of co-construction of visual or written information attached to a product. In this case, the result is labeling. We also refer to *mention* or *allegation*, terms that are in line with a legal approach to terminology.

5 The NA'Stras project (from September 2021 to February 2023) aims to identify, describe and categorize digital devices related to food, and to explain their influence on the links between producers and consumers, in Strasbourg and the Bas-Rhin region. The aim is to gain a better understanding of how digital technologies can be used to promote the consumption and production of healthy, sustainable and local food. In this context, the aim of this article, associated with Action 1 and Action 2 of the NA'Stras project, is to identify, describe and categorize digital tools, as conceived and presented by their designers. More specifically, the focus here is on the descriptive and standard messages conveyed by the bearers through their devices and discourses, as well as the relationships that these actors and objects maintain with one another. The Phyt'Info project (November 2021 to July 2024), which examines the ways in which digital communication contributes to the dissemination and promotion of more ecological practices, focuses on the issue of reducing the use of plant protection products. The NA'Stras and Phyt'Info projects share a common ambition, that of reporting on the ways in which these devices are deployed and the visions of quality they promote. They therefore share the objective of critically reading the process of co-construction of information and the modalities of access to product information, at a time when they promise to facilitate the linkages of market relations between producers and consumers. News from the NA'Stras and Phyt'Info projects can be found at: https://numali.unistra.fr/.

digital intermediaries co-construct the link between producers and consumers, in the light of an economy of quality (Karpik 1989) and an economy of packaging (Cochoy 2002).

2.2.1. *Why communicate about pesticides?*

To begin with, we need to look at the literature that defines "quality". When we talk about the intermediaries that smooth relations between producers and consumers, what are we actually talking about? Labels, certifications, ingredient lists, origins, nutritional declarations, scores, environmental impacts, social impacts, etc. When it comes to filling their food baskets at the store, consumers make choices supported by information systems (Cochoy 2002; Laurent and Mallard 2020). The abundance of decision-making tools at the consumer's disposal has led to fears of an increase in market transparency, due to information asymmetry (Akerlof 1970), or a waste of consumers' cognitive resources, due to a lack (economy) of attention (Goldhaber 1997). Digital mediations are being deployed in market spaces, with the success of mobile apps, in particular as a "new software format" (Morris and Murray 2018). In these "marketplaces", the process of filling the physical basket is represented by a digital basket (icon). The consumer who fills their basket is defined as the guarantor of sustainability. Digital transition and ecological transition are considered together, with the principle of a committed consumer at their core. Therefore, in a context where the co-construction of a new consumer through marketing (Cova and Cova 2009) gives rise to the fictional figure of a sustainable consumer (Beuscart et al. 2020) who is responsible for regulating markets, the digital mediations that equip and participate in "governing conducts" (Dubuisson-Quellier 2016) or more specifically in guiding the food choices of this "consumer-actor", seem to increase their influence on production as well as consumption practices (Chiffoleau et al. 2018). The discourses of the digital actors we interviewed[6] are meaningful: in response to an informational landscape that would render the markets transparent and fail to stimulate the adoption of practices (more precisely here, food) that are said to be healthy, sustainable and local, digital operators intend to position themselves as facilitators of the relationship between producers and consumers. This article examines the ways in which this simplification of market relations is created, between defining food "quality" and building consumer confidence.

The motive for communicating about pesticides certainly finds part of its answer in sociological and information literature, as well as communication science literature, as it looks at changes in the information ecosystem. Recent works set a context, increasing media coverage of the effects of plant protection products

6 There are 15 of them (see Table 2.2).

(Boudet et al. 2020; Botero 2021), with the shift from political agenda-setting, notably in the context of the Grenelle de l'environnement (2007), to media agenda-setting, with an initial time frame (2008–2016) that "pays particular attention to damage to biodiversity" and a second time frame (2017–2020) that "opens onto health scandals and lawsuits" (Botero 2021, p. 110). What emerges from this is an evolution in the "social life" (Appadurai 1988) of the object and, more specifically here, the highlighting of the problems of market arrangements and externalities presented by economic activities (Callon 1998).

2.2.2. *How can we communicate about pesticides?*

While the question of "why" more readily admits the categorical aspect of pesticides, the limited practical aspect of "how" is more versatile. We suggest approaching it by examining the contribution of digital mediations that equip the consumer decision-making process. The usefulness of focusing on digital mediations is justified at a time when the number and use of these devices are increasing, and when they seem to be influencing both production and consumption practices, in particular by supporting greater sustainability of relationships within agri-food systems (Chiffoleau et al. 2018).

A critical reading of the ways in which information is co-constructed to enhance value through the reduction of pesticide use will be carried out in three stages, using three methods:

– A general description of the process by which digital operators define food "quality", with a particular focus on reducing the use of phytosanitary products as a quality characteristic. This work is based on an identification and characterization of the digital devices involved through statistical processing (see section 2.2).

– A reading of the representations of food quality and the intentions expressed by the actors who use these digital tools. This understanding is based on material from semi-structured interviews with representatives of devices that have been previously identified and analyzed (see section 2.3).

– A case study of the Zéro résidu de pesticides (Zero Pesticide Residue) and Planet-score labels, which use the term "pesticide" as a promotional argument. This observation is based on an analysis of gray literature, and an examination of logos and packaging (see section 2.4).

2.3. Commitments to monitoring the use of plant protection products in the definition of food "quality"

When describing the process of presentation, representation and qualification of food "quality" by digital operators, the entry point used is digital socio-technical tools (here, as digital devices), and therefore the actors and relationships embedded in it, which equips consumers and plays a part in their choices. A first phase of research, attached to the NA'Stras project, consisted of locating and identifying the digital tools that link producers and consumers of healthy, sustainable and local food accessible in the territories involved in the study (Bas-Rhin and Occitanie)[7]. To characterize these digital tools, we developed an analysis grid that applies the same reading and content characterization method to each device identified.

2.3.1. *Method for identifying digital devices for guiding food choice*

The inventory of existing tools was carried out by strata and aggregation of different methods[8]. Following this census, a more selective sorting was made, using rigorous selection criteria. Four criteria determined the selection of devices to be retained for analysis:

– Thematic criteria, with the principle of a device that provides information on the conditions for healthy, sustainable and local food.

– Geographical criteria, with a focus on tools that are accessible to the inhabitants of Occitanie and/or Bas-Rhin. To be selected, consumers in the Occitanie and Bas-Rhin regions must be able to benefit from the potential offered by the device.

7 Last grid update: April 2022.

8 A first application involves an extended search with keyword queries on the Google search engine (e.g. "buy organic", "buy local", "buy short distance" or "digital tools for farmers"). This initial survey brought devices to light that belong to our exploratory field, as well as directory sites and articles dealing with healthy, sustainable and local food issues and referring to the tools in question. A second method of investigation extends the initial queries by using hyperlinks that facilitate passage from one relevant site to the next. Visits to platforms such as "Bienvenue à la ferme", "Frais et local" or "Acheter à la source" have proved to be particularly productive in providing links to partner sites or sites operating in the same field. A third stratum is based on contacts established with researchers in Strasbourg, Toulouse and Paris to share resources. This is a time-consuming task, given the care and attention required, but it was necessary in order to acquire an initial list of almost 140 devices.

– Economic criteria, with mediation partly aimed at end consumers. Devices that only concern producers, distributors or manufacturers are therefore excluded.

– Digital centrality criteria, with digital mediation at the heart of the player's commercial approach. Digital devices that have been developed as an improvement to an existing, central, non-digital offer are therefore excluded.

A list of 55 devices was drawn up, based on the criteria presented above.

2.3.2. *Statistical treatment*

The analysis grid is designed to translate descriptive and analytical categories into variables and thus takes the form of a series of codes designed to be as close as possible to the data observed, as well as to limit preconceptions and other interpretation bias[9]. For the most part, these codes consist of dichotomous variables (which only have two attributes: true or false), enabling a greater variety of statistical treatments.

The 55 devices selected are subjected to statistical treatment, including 62 variables.

2.3.2.1. *Variables related to the qualification of food quality by digital devices*

We will concentrate here on describing one particular set of variables, the inventory of elements used by the devices to define food quality. By qualification, we mean all of the attributes explicitly mentioned (on the first page of the mediation) by the devices as arguments for enhancing the value of the food products and/or producers concerned. The list is exhaustive, and includes references to organic farming, local produce, nutritional value, affordability, practicality, consideration of environmental issues, social justice, ethics, waste management (frugality, sorting, recycling), short distance, seasonality, tasting pleasure, conviviality and, last but not least, reducing the use of plant protection products.

A first statistical treatment consists of a flat sorting of all of these characteristics. This analysis highlights the frequency of the variables.

Dealing with the reduction in the use of phytosanitary products requires taking a brief but preliminary look at the indications that mark the quality of food production and consumption. This examination is based on a broader understanding of the

9 For example, being organic is a different representation of quality from that of respect for the environment, or nutritional value (the characteristics attributed to organic farming can be ranked in different hierarchies by the players involved).

issues surrounding communication between players involved in the co-construction of healthy, sustainable food. One of the aims of the study is to identify what distinguishes (or not) quality labels promoting the reduction of plant protection products from other indices of food quality, because when these devices are conceived and developed, their designers participate in defining and setting the qualities of goods, in qualifying products[10] and, in so doing, they promote measures designed to capture their attention (Cochoy 2004) and divert these message recipients[11] from their course. More specifically, they focus on presenting, representing and qualifying (Barrey et al. 2000; Cochoy 2002; Laurent and Mallard 2020) healthy, sustainable and local food quality, and on recruiting (Akrich et al. 1998) the actors concerned in this qualification of food quality[12].

---

10 While the term *qualification* more traditionally refers to the assessment of professional skills, it was not until the early 1980s that the issue of quality and qualification became part of the study of the product market. From an analytical point of view, quality is studied as a co-production between producers and users. There is an abundance of academic literature on the issues surrounding the presentation, representation and qualification of products on the market stage. Addressing this literature implies taking an interest in the market devices that support exchange and help it to take place. As we place these devices at the heart of our analysis, we are interested in the process of co-constructing legitimate reference systems for product quality, qualification and re-qualification, carried out by players on both the supply and demand sides. Indeed, when we speak of healthy, sustainable and local food, we are involved in a process of elaborating these notions and consolidating standardization. We are therefore attentive to this co-construction and wish to highlight the relationships between categorization of devices and definition of healthy, sustainable and local food. What are the elements that define quality? In line with the themes addressed, and after examining the sites, the qualities listed here refer to organic, local, nutritional, money-saving, practical, environmental, social, waste and sorting, short distance, seasonality, reduced use of plant protection products, pleasure and satisfaction.

11 Very practically, a consumer moves around the Web in search of information and, if a message resonates with them, they will stop browsing and immerse themselves in reading paragraphs on a particular site. For the market player, building this match between the message and the hypothetical consumer is a major challenge, such as the skillful path to dialogue and gaining the individual's attention. Historically, these dispositions have been sought on the side of interest (influenced by the economic tradition) or habit (influenced by the sociological tradition), but this duality has been challenged and has opened up to a plurality of levers. What are the dispositions we will be questioning here in the context of our current investigation? In line with the themes addressed, the dispositions listed here are interest, respect for the environment, ethics (in the sense of a social and supportive consideration of the players), respect for the body (in the nutritional sense), pleasure (in the gustatory, as well as satisfactory sense) and playfulness (which here is humor, amused curiosity).

12 Since the seminal work of Akerlof (1970) and Stiglitz (1987), and in particular the work of Karpik (1989), we have been aware of the importance of identification and assessment in

There is a very clear distinction here: the devices do not mention pesticides. Local (54.5% of devices explicitly refer to it), social justice (49.1% of devices explicitly refer to it), environmental issues (40% of devices explicitly refer to it), short distance (40% of devices explicitly refer to it) or the centrality of the AB label (36.4% of devices explicitly refer to it) are mentioned on the very first page (home page). This page, which is immediately visible to consumers when they log on to the site, gives them an initial appreciation of the content of the mediation, but no reference to the use of plant protection products is made on any of the devices examined.

Characteristics	Usage by the device	Nonuse by the device
Organic farming	20 (36.4%)	35 (63.6%)
Local	30 (54.5%)	25 (45.5%)
Nutritional benefits	15 (27.3%)	40 (72.7%)
Financial savings	6 (10.9%)	49 (89.1%)
Practicality	17 (30.9%)	38 (69.1%)
Environmental issues	22 (40%)	33 (60%)
Social justice, ethics	27 (49.1%)	28 (50.9%)
Waste management	4 (7.3%)	51 (92.7%)
Short distance	22 (40%)	33 (60%)
Seasonality	7 (12.7%)	48 (87.3%)
Tasting pleasure	15 (27.3%)	40 (72.7%)
Satisfaction	7 (12.7%)	48 (87.3%)
Reducing the use of plant protection products	0	0

Table 2.1. *Frequency of quality characteristics explicitly used by digital devices*

---

reducing the uncertainty required to establish an exchange. The aim of identification is to stabilize a product's quality attributes. The importance of the assessment work that follows identification stems from the realization that, although identification is necessary, it is not sufficient when it comes to overcoming uncertainty. This "overcoming" is made possible by the work involved in defining the mechanisms of judgment and commitment (and therefore of trust) that support the completion of the transaction. If the intermediaries that equip consumers' cognition do not help reconfigure the information and representation of food quality, as well as the relationships between the aforementioned players, the problem of the "proper" functioning of markets arises (Cochoy 2002; Dubuisson-Quellier and Neuville 2003; François 2011).

2.4. The role of plant protection product use in quality assessment using digital devices

The references to plant protection products are undeniably insignificant and therefore meaningless as the subject seems to be overlooked. If we venture beyond this first page, four sites nevertheless refer to it. The very limited use of the phytosanitary argument made by digital operators is all the more surprising in a context where the appropriation of arguments related to healthy, local and sustainable eating is otherwise abundant. Our analysis of the digital devices studied leads us to consider the existence of a socio-technical lock-in, in other words, the idea of "forces and power relations that translate into forms that sometimes 'become irreversible', at least for a time" (Callon and Ferrary 2006, p. 38). The principle of socio-technical lock-in is an initial cross-sectional hypothesis of the Phyt'Info project. As a reminder, following on from the Grenelle de l'environnement, the Ecophyto 2018 plan introduced in September 2008 sets the (unmet) target of reducing the use of plant protection products in agriculture by 50% by 2018. This plan, steered by the French Ministry of Agriculture, prescribes an approach that primarily relies on the knowledge and expertise of technicians from chambers of agriculture and technical institutes, and makes research and farmer training a priority. In the wake of the Ecophyto plan's failure, and in parallel with its evolution, assessments of its actions and related research are highlighting areas for progress, including consideration of the socio-technical bottlenecks that stand in the way of a desired ecological transition (Guichard et al. 2017). This is a source of local controversy in agricultural policies that can take many forms and generate results with varying degrees of success, with a transition that is "marginal in practice" (Pahun 2020, thesis summary). So for us, it is a question of acknowledging the existence of an absence, a lock-in that involves the process of characterizing food quality. Our analysis will focus less on the existence of this lock-in than on the reasons for the discreet use of claims related to plant protection products.

2.4.1. *Information "lock-in": interviews with representatives of the devices*

The reasons for these exclusions were investigated in a second phase of research, which involved semi-structured interviews with a sample of representatives of the devices that had been previously identified and analyzed.

Device (description)	Name of the holder (anonymized)
Site (private)	Julien – Industry Manager
Platform (private)	Lena – Co-founder
Site (private)	Marc and Faustine – Co-founders
Directory/map (association)	Philippe – Communications Manager
Directory/map (association)	Delphine – Development Manager
Platform (private)	Christine – Founder
Directory/map (association)	Hans – Manager
Application (association)	Maxime – Co-founder
Application (private)	Pierre – Founder
Platform (private)	Pierre – Founder
Platform (private)	Laura – Development Manager
Directory/map (association)	Adeline – Communications Manager
Directory/map (association)	Fanny – Manager
Site (public actor)	Juliette – Team manager
Directory/map (association)	Dominique – Volunteer

Table 2.2. *(Anonymized) list of digital device representatives that were interviewed*

The questions are: what can we learn from a cross-analysis in terms of the ways in which devices are structured and the discourses of the designers of these same devices? What do the interviewees have to say about the modest role played by the use of plant protection products in the qualification of food quality?

"So really, each to their own, and that is why it is not easy to find a definite and radical position on the issue, as (x – name of platform). That is why we have chosen to be somewhere in between, in other words, to ask producers on (x – name of platform) to reduce their use of plant protection products as much as possible, but without forcing them to do so, and without setting any limits, so it is up to everyone's free interpretation. […] For some people it is an important point, particularly our partner, and she was the one who really wanted to make it clear, and I think it is a good thing because it is linked to the Earth's balance" (Lena).

"The difficulty we have, in fact, is that communicating on a reduction… Communicating on a suppression is very easy, but communicating on a reduction implies that there is a use. And today, these are words… 'phytosanitary' is a very technical word, but 'pesticide' is a word that can no longer be used when talking to consumers about food. […] We do not put too much emphasis on it, and we are trying to find the right ways of communicating so that we are both transparent and so that this transparency does not actually do us any harm. [...] In any case, it is the choice of the agricultural sector as a whole. It is their choice to overlook this part because it is easier, in fact, even when we are talking about organic farming, because 90, 95, 99% of consumers think that a product with the organic label is necessarily phyto-free" (Julien).

Box 2.1. *Plant protection products, a (dis)qualification of quality*

Two difficulties are mentioned: one in adopting a clearly defined position on the use (or nonuse) of plant protection products and, by extension, an awkwardness in talking about them, resulting in fragmented communication. Here, we find ourselves in the difficult position of stabilizing scientifically legitimate characteristics that obstruct the validation of exchange rules. With regard to the obstacles to positioning, Lena describes a form of blurring that leaves an interstice and regulation, which are left to the arbitration of each individual. She goes on to point out that the reference, made on site, to the reduction of plant protection products is essentially the result of a partner who is sensitive to arguments related to environmental protection. With regard to the obstacles to assertive communication, Julien highlights two negative considerations that are mutually reinforcing, namely that praising reduction means making its presence felt, and admitting its presence means potentially upsetting consumer expectations (purchases). A consensus was also reached on the silence of "the agricultural sector as a whole". If we mention the hypothesis of communication with mediation providers who could legitimately take advantage of this provision, another form of silence is described.

"In fact, we always remind people that all organic products are free from synthetic phytosanitary chemicals, so there you go. However, we do not insist on it any more than that" (Philippe).

"Plant protection is a double-edged sword. For organic farming, it is a very solid guarantee that no chemical inputs are used. At the same time, it does not mean that natural inputs aren't used. And there's a fear among those involved in organic farming that, one day, there will be a scandal involving a natural product, and that this will shatter the image that organic farming does not use chemicals. It is an extremely sensitive subject, and it is the main point of attack for those who protest organic farming, who always say: 'but organic farming uses inputs'" (Fanny).

"It is in our name, (x – platform name). [...] I had a gem this week, someone told me: 'I had a good look but I do not know if all your products are organic, it would be good to write it on each product.' I'm saying that as long as it is labeled *organic*, you do not need to write it on every product. The labels are displayed for each producer, so that was this week's little gem. We are a community of people who do not want to ask ourselves: 'oh, is this organic or isn't it?'. They know that at the very least, it is organic" (Christine).

Box 2.2. *Organic: silence on the plant protection argument*

It is curious to note that even the players who are in a position to use the highly regulated use of plant protection products as a marketing argument do not think it necessary to emphasize this claim. This argument is considered to be sufficiently emphasized in the labeling of products or in the names of operators. Above all, a certain fear that criticism of the use of natural plant protection products will nonetheless be exercised curbs any hypothetical willingness to communicate on these subjects. This dual blockage invites us to question the a priori antagonistic aspect of the use of plant protection products. An entry through the "economy of the signal", or an entry through the notions of meanings, of symbols (Baudrillard 1970), which are intrinsic to the functioning of markets (and more specifically in the case of food markets), provide initial keys to interpretation. In the 1950s, advertising became more rationalized, focusing in particular on motivations (Dichter 1961). In terms of form, it sought to play on "meanings" and symbols (Baudrillard 1970), equipping consumers with cognitive tools (Denis and Pontille 2010) that helped influence practices. Here, the controversies associated with plant protection products are of concern to all actors, who prefer not to deal with them, whether or not this aspect can be an asset. There is an understanding here of how crucial the second sequence of media agenda-setting is, to recall a second timescale (2017–2020) that "opens onto health scandals and lawsuits" (Botero 2021, p. 110). This is one of the singularities of our aim, which questions the modalities of communication, in a context of market tensions and movements of the actors who constitute it. We can see how difficult it is to value goods associated with controversial products and contested markets (Steiner and Trespeuch 2015), or at least the "relevant market" (Geiger et al. 2014). Thinking in terms of a contested market means looking at goods whose marketing raises controversies, in this case the controversy imposed by the association between fruit and vegetables, and the pesticides associated with their production and consumption. Thinking in terms of the relevant market means facing a market that generates fears. Actors in the market recoil when faced with a sensitive subject. Respondents are also keen to promote a renewal of communication, in other words, the establishment of dialogue and translation, and the reconfiguration of symbols that are currently locked in.

"Regarding the development of organic farming [...] as there were these double-digit growth rates, no one asked themselves whether they should communicate or invest resources. Today, it is clear that we need to start explaining things to consumers again if we want the organic sector to continue to develop" (Fanny).

"I think there is a communication problem. 'Bleu Blanc Coeur' and 'Zéro pesticide'... 'Zéro pesticide' succeeded in communicating, whereas we were quietly sailing along on all our achievements and there was a lack... well... of communication. I sincerely believe that is part of it too" (Adeline).

Box 2.3. *Is it necessary to break the silence?*

2.5. Initiatives to "unlock information": the case of Zéro résidu de pesticides and Planet-score

Despite the various difficulties involved in providing information on the use or nonuse of plant protection products, some actors have chosen to use the term *pesticides* in their information messages. These claims, which are few in number, are made by the Nouveaux Champs collective[13] (Zéro résidu de pesticides), the Alliance Nature et Saveurs[14] (cultivated without pesticides), the Demain la Terre association[15] (the "without" approaches, in other words, "cultivated without synthetic pesticides" and "without pesticide residue detected"), and the Institut technique de l'agriculture biologique[16] (Planet-score). We took a closer look at two of them: Zéro résidu de pesticides and Planet-score. The Nouveaux Champs collective, which bears the Zéro résidu de pesticides label, caught our attention because of its pioneering role. The timescales of the initiative are consistent with the observations described above regarding the sequencing of the media agenda of references to pesticides (Botero 2021). The Zéro résidu de pesticides label was rolled out in 2018, in an information landscape, lacking in references to the use of plant protection products. As for Planet-score, it is the environmental label that is most closely involved in digital communication strategies, with its collaboration with the Omie brand in particular, making it a particularly relevant subject of analysis for us. The cardinal principle of both is to think of the use of meaningful terminology as an information asset, contrary to the popular doxa revealed among digital operators. What we speak of here is a resemantization that wagers "positive naming" (Libaert and Allard-Huver 2014), or more precisely, that has been made positive, by the overt use of negative naming. What, then, can we learn from mere information in these media? Referring to an analysis in terms of certification, the commercial equipment for cognition, there are two paths to follow here: the transfer of actors' responsibilities and the diversification of indicators.

2.5.1. *Zéro résidu de pesticides (Zero pesticide residues)*

The Nouveaux Champs collective describes itself as:

> A citizen movement of French producers – voluntary actors in the transformation of our country's agriculture. Committed to human and environmental progress, we defend healthy eating for all. Today, we

13 The Nouveaux Champs collective represents 60 companies and 600 producers.

14 Initiated by three cooperatives (Prince de Bretagne, Savéol and Solarenn) representing 176 producers.

15 An association, under French law 1901, of producers of fresh and processed fruit and vegetables.

16 French Technical Institute for Organic Farming.

> are able to offer a wide range of foods guaranteed to contain 'zero pesticide residues' in the fresh fruit and vegetable, frozen food, dried fruit, juice, pasta and wine sections[17].

The label was developed in 2017 and applied to products at the start of 2018, a date that enabled actors to take hold of an emerging media issue. The approach thus bets "on a model of reassurance by offering a guarantee to the consumer. The agriculture of proof (or of results) is a source of commitment. It is a response to defending good eating for all, a civic commitment"[18]. In terms of impact, whether it be the popularity of the logo or the effect it has on the sales of the products concerned, there are a number of influences to be observed. The Zéro résidu de pesticides logo is one of 11 symbols of quality whose awareness, reputation, attention and trust were tested by Agence bio and the CSA Institute[19]. The Zéro résidu de pesticides logo was seen by 50% of those questioned, 36% were aware of it (47% in Occitanie, 36% in Grand Est) and 80% of those questioned trusted it (80% in Occitanie, 76% in Grand Est). When shopping in-store, 71% of consumers are aware of this symbol of quality (64% in Occitanie, 76% in Grand Est). From the economic rationality perspective, a quarter of French people have bought Zéro résidu de pesticides products, and 36 items are currently labeled, representing 200 available references, including 15 wine references. A 9% increase in sales by value between 2020 and 2021 was announced by the Nouveaux Champs collective in a press briefing on February 23, 2022. On July 26, 2021, the Zéro résidu de pesticides approach was awarded level 2 HVE certification by the French Ministry of Agriculture.

In Figure 2.1, we can see a tray of cocktail tomatoes marketed by Les paysans de Rougeline, founding members of the Nouveaux Champs collective.

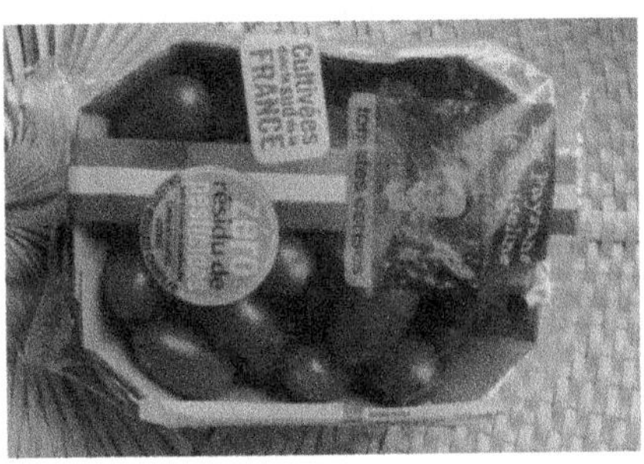

Figure 2.1. *Tray of cherry tomatoes marketed by Les paysans de Rougeline. For a color section of this figure, see www.iste.co.uk/botero/pesticides.zip*

17 See: www.nouveaux-champs.fr/ [accessed September 20, 2022].

18 Page 27 of the press kit. Available at: www.nouveaux-champs.fr/wp-content/uploads/2020/02/dp_collectif_nouveaux_champs_v27.pdf [Accessed September 20, 2022].

19 Consumer barometer and perception of organic products in France. Agence Bio/CSA. January 2022.

2.5.1.1. *Shifting responsibilities*

In terms of its shape, the Zéro résidu de pesticides claim is a green, round label. The color categories can be noticed, with "Zéro" and "pesticides" published in white, and "résidue de" (residue) as well as "dans les limites de quantification" (within quantification limits), "cahier des charges contrôlé" (controlled specifications), and "collectif Nouveaux Champs" (Nouveaux Champs collective) published in black. Note the size scale, with "Zéro", "pesticides", "résidue", "collectif Nouveaux Champs", "cahier des charges contrôlé" and "dans les limites de quantification" in descending order. The graphic used shows that "Zéro pesticides" has a larger profile than "résidue de", "collectif Nouveaux Champs" and "cahier des charges contrôlé", with "dans les limites de quantification" being the smallest.

In terms of content, the specifications drawn up by the Nouveaux Champs collective are in line with Interfel's recommendations guide on the use of negative claims concerning pesticides and pesticide residues in the fresh fruit and vegetable sector. More specifically, the Zéro résidu de pesticides program guarantees consumers the absence of residues at the consumption stage, within the limit of quantification[20]. The specifications do not currently include a ban on the use of chemical fertilizers, but committed producers must verify that no residues have been generated during processing. In fact, "zero" does not mean absence, but rather the possible presence of traces below a threshold defined by the limits of quantification.

In addition to complying with the Interfel recommendation guidelines[21], the Nouveaux Champs collective's Zéro résidu de pesticides (zero pesticide residue) label is a response to the difficulty of communicating the reduction principle mentioned above. "Zero" suggests absence, elimination, and shifts responsibility from the pesticide in its projection, to the pesticide residue detected at the end of production. If it is the residue that is responsible, then its absence (or possibly its presence below a defined minimum threshold) removes the fruit or vegetable from the controversial product that disqualifies it. The message has a dual impact: in substance, through the appropriation of the term "residue", associated with a limit of quantification that allows the use of the term "zero"; on the form, with a kind of alienation of the same term, carried by a play on sizes and colors in the graphics. In essence, this inspires a change in a statement that could be "traces of pesticides within the limit of quantification" into a perceived "zero pesticides" statement. We

20 Smallest value that can be quantified by laboratories with "acceptable" accuracy.

21 Guide available on the Interfel website. Available at: www.interfel.com/recherche/type-documentation/?s=all%C3%A9gations%20pesticides [Accessed October 4, 2022].

thus find an unlocking of information that relies on the shift of the controversial aspect and opens the way to a third agricultural path[22].

2.5.1.2. *A combination of evaluation devices*

However, it is worth highlighting the national and regional bias represented by the French colors here, with the words "cultivées dans le sud de la France" ("grown in the south of France"), and the personalization (photo of a grower). The commitments of the producers involved in the Nouveaux Champs collective program and the Zéro résidu de pesticides label are shown on the side of the packaging, which is made from recyclable cardboard.

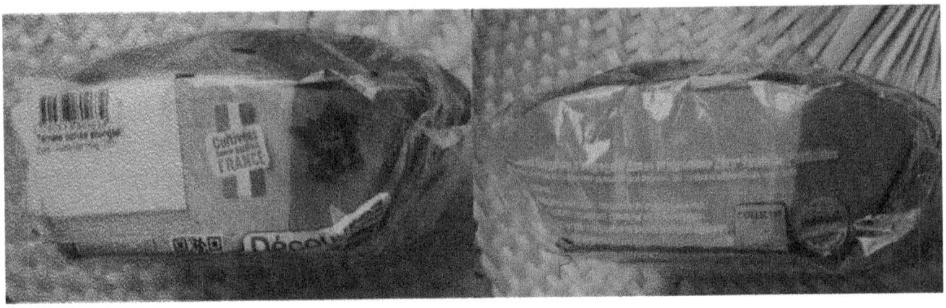

Figure 2.2. *Sides of the tray marketed by Les paysans de Rougeline. For a color version of this figure, see www.iste.co.uk/botero/pesticides.zip*

Identifying these elements highlights the associations that make up the market layout. In fact, the evaluation system is based on a number of features which, when combined, reinforce consumer trust and facilitate product assessment. Personalization through the use of a producer's face, reference to the locality (national and regional), the list of commitments, the reduction of plastic packaging, are all signs that structure a superposition of legitimate quality characteristics, play on consumers' supposed

22 The notion of a third agricultural path appears in the Nouveaux Champs press kit (p. 20). Available at: www.nouveaux-champs.fr/wp content/uploads/2020/02/dp_collectif_nouveaux_champs_v27.pdf [Accessed September 20, 2022]. This term is often used by Bioline by InVivo (one of the four partners of the business club created in September 2021, with which the Nouveaux Champs collective is associated). This notion of the third path is also used by the Demain la Terre, Bleu Blanc Cœur, Vignerons en développement durable and CRC® associations, which have created a "third path collective" (see: www.troisiemevoieagricole.com/). The third path is defined as follows: today, there is not **one** form of agriculture, but **many** different forms of agriculture that coexist. "Alongside conventional and organic farming, there is a third path, where producers in each agricultural sector work within the same logic of environmental, economic, social and societal responsibility".

dispositions, and support the product assessment process. Ultimately, the Zéro résidu de pesticides claim should not be considered alone, while failing to consider the system in its entirety, in other words, as a multi-criteria layout.

This multi-criteria approach can be found in a renewed form with Planet-score.

2.5.2. *Planet-score*

Planet-score is an environmental label developed by the French Institute of Organic Agriculture and Food (ITAB), and its partners Sayari[23] and Very Good future[24]. This proposal for display is in response to a call for projects (and specifications) to take part in an experiment led by ADEME and the French Ministry of Ecological Transition and Territorial Cohesion, in order to define an environmental display for food products (currently in the assessment phase)[25].

2.5.2.1. *Legislative framework for environmental labeling*

The Planet-score approach is part of a broader context (food and nonfood), relating to environmental labeling, and is in line with the following:

– Environmental information for consumers, as defined in Article 90 of the LTECV (French law on energy transition and green growth). "In order to guarantee the quality of the environmental information made available to consumers, producers who voluntarily make an environmental communication or claim concerning their products are required to jointly make available the main environmental characteristics of these products"[26].

– The recommendations of the French Ministry of Ecological Transition and Territorial Cohesion, which provide a framework for environmental labeling aimed

23 Sayari is a consulting firm specializing in the environmental field, founded in 2018. On the site's home page (see: www.sayari.co/), the motto is "Foster your business. Nurture the planet".

24 Very Good Future is a consulting firm created at the end of 2019. It supports project leaders and presents itself on its website (see: www.verygoodfuture.com/) as the "accelerator of projects with impact for more sustainable agriculture and food" [Accessed September 20, 2022].

25 See: www.expertises.ademe.fr/economie-circulaire/consommer-autrement/passer-a-laction/reconnaitre-produit-plus-respectueux-lenvironnement/dossier/laffichage-environnemental/affichage-environnemental-secteur-alimentaire-experimentation-20202021 [Accessed September 21, 2022].

26 The aim is to provide a framework for environmental claims, with a multi-criteria vision, and to control greenwashing. See: www.ecologie.gouv.fr/laffichage-environnemental-des-produits-et-des-services-hors-alimentaire/ [Accessed September 20, 2022].

at informing consumers' purchasing decisions through relevant, transparent information. They are specified on the French Ministry's website:

- separate presentation of results for each environmental indicator;

- a very compact presentation that can be directly applied to product packaging or shelves, in the form of an overall grade with a letter grade of A, B, C, D or E (A being the best grade);

- an aggregated version can be used as a first reading level, and should then refer to the details of the indicators;

- the results specific to each product are first accounted for through a limited number of environmental impact indicators (generally between three and five indicators), and greenhouse gas emissions are systematically considered[27].

– Law no. 2020-105 of February 10, 2020 on the fight against waste and the circular economy, known as the AGEC law (anti-waste for a circular economy) includes a title II on "consumer information" (articles 12–29)[28].

– The Climate and resilience law 2021-1104 of August 22, 2021, which combats climate change and builds resilience to its effects. In particular Article 2 on consumer information, environmental display and its experimentation[29].

2.5.2.2. *Framing the Planet-score environmental display proposal*

The methodology presented by the ITAB as part of its environmental display proposal[30] mainly uses, as stipulated in Article 15.1[31] of Law No. 2020-105 of February 10, 2020 on the fight against waste and the circular economy, the life cycle

27 See: www.ecologie.gouv.fr/laffichage-environnemental-des-produits-et-des-services-hors-alimentaire/ [Accessed September 20, 2022].

28 Decree 2022-748 of April 29, 2022 implements Article 13 of the AGEC law, making it compulsory for consumers to be informed of certain environmental characteristics of products on the market, and provides a framework for the environmental claims made on them.

29 See: www.legifrance.gouv.fr/jorf/article_jo/JORFARTI000043956979 [Accessed September 20, 2022].

30 See: https://www.bio-centre.org/index.php/a-la-une/551-planet-score-pour-un-affichage-environnemental-des-produits-alimentaires.

31 Article 15.1: "A voluntary environmental, or environmental and social, display device is hereby instituted. It is intended to provide consumers with environmental, or environmental and social, criteria information on a good, service or category of goods or services, based primarily on a life cycle analysis".

analysis (ACV) method[32], and this is based on the Agribalyse agricultural and food products database[33]. However, as stated in ADEME's call for tender: "Projects will be primarily based on life cycle analysis, but project leaders are invited to use complementary indicators as well". This invitation echoes the "limitations and need for evolution of the ACV methodology", pointed out on the Agribalyse documentary site[34], and thus the work in progress aimed at developing ACV indicators to improve the current framework, which does not take all environmental impacts into account. In response to the Agribalyse 3.0 database published on the ADEME website in September 2020, the ITAB questioned the limits of Agribalyse data in a December 14, 2020 document entitled: Questions on the relevance of Agribalyse 3.0 data for the environmental assessment of agricultural products and the environmental labeling of food products[35].

To meet the specifications of the call for tenders and the recommendations of the experiment's scientific council, the proposal from the ITAB and its partners is based on the ACV foundation and adds complementary indicators to express environmental impacts that are poorly covered by the ACV.

2.5.2.3. *Consumer information: the Planet-score visual*

The Planet-score environmental label has a synthetic, interpretative and colorful format. It consists of a color scale ranging from dark green to dark orange, with the letters A to E distributed on it. The aggregate score for a product is used to assign a letter and show the rating on the scale. In addition to this aggregate score, three additional indicators are clearly expressed (pesticides, biodiversity, climate) and are marked on a grading scale, without a letter, but reproducing the color codes mentioned. The value for each of the three indicators is represented by a cursor

32 The ACV method is used for quantifying a product's impact on the environment throughout its life cycle (multi-stage), taking into account several environmental issues (multi-criteria). It is governed by the ISO 14044 standard and is used internationally by the scientific community, the private sector and public authorities. Sixteen indicators are provided (indicators recommended by the European Commission's Product Environmental Footprint project, which aims to define and assess the environmental footprint of products – a European regulation is expected). For each product category, a single score is calculated on the basis of the 16 indicators.

33 Agribalyse is a program initiated in 2013 that provides a database for the environmental analysis of agricultural and food products.

34 See: https://doc.agribalyse.fr/documentation [Accessed September 24, 2022].

35 Original French version: *Questions sur la pertinence des données Agribalyse 3.0 pour l'évaluation environnementale des produits agricoles et l'affichage environnemental des produits alimentaires*. See: https://www.cade-environnement.org/wp-content/uploads/2020/12/Communiqu%C3%A9-ITAB-rapport-Agribalyse-20201214-v.pdf [Accessed September 24, 2022].

(circle) at the center of one of the five colored segments. In addition, there is a pictogram related to farming conditions (for farm-raised products or foods containing farm-raised products), an indicator which, however, is not included in the calculation of the score. In a way, this display combines a single score (through an aggregated rating) with multi-criteria information by adding additional indicators.

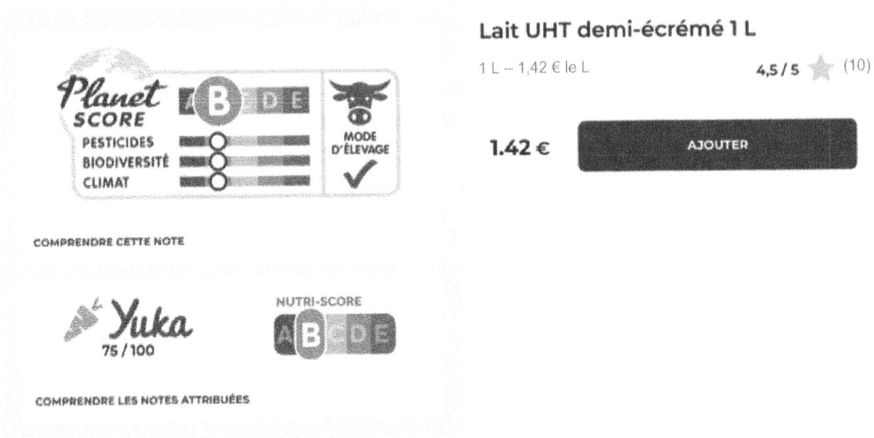

Figure 2.3. *Planet-score visual of pesticides, biodiversity and climate (combined with Yuka and Nutri-score ratings) for 1 L of 2% milk (on the Omie website). For a color version of this figure, see www.iste.co.uk/botero/pesticides.zip*

Two levers need to be highlighted: the association between the multiple clear criteria for the label and the homogeneity of the associated labels.

Considering Planet-score alone as an independent sign of quality prompts us to focus on the diversification of indicators. Following on from a consumer study carried out on a sample of 1,000 people, representative of the French population (cross-referenced with a qualitative in-store survey), three key results are highlighted by the ITAB and Very Good Future in their various communications[36]: consumer appeal for evocative and transparent terms, as well as for multi-criteria claims, and consumer preference[37] for the Planet-score (as opposed to an aggregate score and a multi-criteria score, which does not use the term "pesticide"). The study

36 See: www.itab.asso.fr/activites/planet-score.php [Accessed September 25, 2022].

37 We recommend looking at the third result, which concludes that consumers prefer the Planet-score visual, in order to suggest that it may be wrong to ask a consumer outside the context of consumption to compare mentions that offer similar information, when the consumer's "qualcul" (Cochoy 2011) instead operates on the principle of associating different information.

asserts that consumers are captured by clarity and plurality, a statement that brings about two hypotheses. The first hypothesis is to consider the use of a terminology that is clear, legible and advantageous, using the term "pesticide" as a source of confidence. Using a term that can potentially be a source of tension within the system would generate trust and reassurance for a wary consumer. While commercial products are silent on the issue of the use of plant protection products, bypassing this fear associated with the controversial product would have a beneficial effect on the consumer's perception of the quality of the approach. The second hypothesis is to think of diversification as a lever for finding the optimum level of reassurance, without resorting to manipulative mechanisms (Beauvois and Joule 1987). Finding the optimal number means improving cognitive efficiency, by linking trust to the number of variables. More precisely, the question of an optimal number of claims is the idea of a number that is managed to avoid cognitive overload, and sufficient to avoid a feeling of transparency. A third hypothesis would be to think of diversification as a lever for decentralizing the consumer's focus, particularly on the controversial term "pesticide". Indeed, thinking of the association of terms means reducing the potential controversy associated with one of them, as the product is not simply a question of whether or not pesticides are used. A fourth hypothesis is to consider the mention of the use of plant protection products as an effective lever for capturing the public's attention. Here, the underlying assumption is that market actors are translating consumers' wishes in line with their own reluctance. The fictitious figure of a consumer invalidating a product that mentions pesticides on its packaging would have been an initially faulty stance, and the term "pesticide" would ultimately be an effective captivating lever.

Furthermore, as part of our study of digital mediations associating certifications or signals, it seems relevant for us to take a situated approach that is more focused on distributed cognition[38] (Hutchins 1993), or at least a composite digital assembly. Considering all of the mentions used on the website of the ITAB partner Omie, and more specifically the Planet-score it uses for all of its products, this prompts us to describe the consumer's complex cognitive equipment. This is complexity offset by a certain homogeneity. Returning to the visual of the Planet-score label proposal (Figure 2.3), we note the common graphic design that unites the Planet-score, the Yuka score and the Nutri-score, with recurring colors, rating and scale, as in path dependency (North 1990; Pierson 2000), which is advantageous here at a time when the Nutri-score, an initial decision to represent hierarchy, guides subsequent choices. Reading, and translation, becomes cognitively easier, and supports multi-criteria information intake. We also note the presence of the score of consumer opinions on the right, as a judgment device, and the price, which does not exclude the possibility of economic calculation.

38 In market spaces with multiple affordances, numerous consumer-support devices populate the space, supporting the skills of the individual.

2.6. Conclusion

From the economics of quality to the economics of packaging, we have traced the definition of quality back to the issue of communication surrounding the use of plant protection products. The first observation is compelling, suggesting that pesticide-specific communication suffers from an information lock-in, linked to the debates surrounding the controversial product, or at least the market concerned. In response, some initiatives have taken the risk of coordinating with the media's focus on the criticisms surrounding the use of pesticides, of qualifying product quality in terms of the reduced use of plant protection products, and of using it as a device that plays on sentiments that are supposedly capable of capturing consumers' attention and diverting them from their trajectory. All we had to do then was observe the ways in which the term "pesticide" was used in the co-construction of the socio-technical labeling system, and the market and cognitive arrangements involved. We hypothesized the following conditions:

– shifting the responsibilities of stakeholders, which transforms the meaning of information for consumers, and in this case, more specifically, communication in terms of deletion;

– diversification, which generates the trust that is essential for market fluidity, when based on optimum reassurance and trust through transparency;

– the association of scores and brands with common designs that identify the quality characteristics while saving the consumer's cognition[39].

2.7. References

Akerlof, G.A. (1970). The market for "lemons": Quality uncertainty and the market mechanism. *The Quarterly Journal of Economics*, 84(3), 488–500.

Akrich, M., Callon, M., Latour, B. (1988). À quoi tient le succès des innovations ? 1. L'art de l'intéressement. 2. Le choix des porte-parole. Gérer et comprendre. *Annales des mines*, 11–12, 4–17, 14–29.

Appadurai, A. (1988). *The Social Life of Things. Commodities in Cultural Perspective*. Cambridge University Press, Cambridge.

Aykut, S.C. and Dahan, A. (2015). *Gouverner le climat : vingt ans de négociations internationales*. Presses de Sciences Po, Paris.

39 All of these hypotheses will be tested as part of the WP4 framework of the Phyt'Info project relating to the analysis of behaviors, in situations of use (focus groups) of digital devices, of consumers in Bas-Rhin, France. The digital navigations of the participants will be followed via ad hoc software.

Barrey, S., Cochoy, F., Dubuisson-Quellier, S. (2000). Designer, packager et merchandiser : trois professionnels pour une même scène marchande. *Sociologie du travail*, 42(3), 457–482.

Baudrillard, J. (1970). *La société de consommation*. Gallimard, Paris.

Beauvois, J.-L. and Joule, R.-V. (1987). *Petit traité de manipulation à l'usage des honnêtes gens*. Presses Universitaires de Grenoble, Grenoble.

Beuscart, J.-B., Peugeot, V., Pharabod, A.-S. (2020). Gouverner numériquement les conduites ? Les technologies de la transition écologique. In *Les technologies et le gouvernement des marchés. Des algorithmes aux biotechnologies*, Kessous, E. and Nau, J.-P. (eds). L'Harmattan, Paris.

Botero, N. (2021). Soustraire l'alimentation du débat sur les pesticides : traitement médiatique d'un problème en une. In *Qu'est-ce que l'on mange ? Les savoirs alimentaires à l'aune des Sciences de l'Information et de la Communication*, Hugol-Gential, C., Badau, E., Michon, D., Parizot, A (eds). Éditions Universitaires de Dijon, Dijon.

Boudet, C., Wallet, F., Thybaud, É. (2020). Pesticides : diversité des sources d'information et effet sur la perception des risques. *Environnement, risques & santé*, 19, 82–89.

Callon, M. (1998). An essay on framing and overflowing: Economic externalities revisited by sociology. *The Sociological Review*, 46(1_suppl), 244–269. doi: 10.1111/j.1467-954X.1998.tb03477.x

Callon, M. and Ferrary, M. (2006). Les réseaux sociaux à l'aune de la théorie de l'acteur-réseau. *Sociologies pratiques*, 2(2), 37–44.

Chiffoleau, Y., Bouré, M., Akermann, G. (2018). Les circuits courts alimentaires à l'heure du numérique : quels enjeux ? Une exploration. *Innovations agronomiques*, 67, 37–47.

Cochoy, F. (2002). *Une sociologie du packaging ou l'âne de Buridan face au marché*. Presses Universitaires de France, Paris.

Cochoy, F. (2004). La captation des publics entre dispositifs et dispositions, ou le petit chaperon rouge revisité. In *La captation des publics : c'est pour mieux te séduire mon client...*. Presses Universitaires du Mirail, Toulouse.

Cochoy, F. (2011). Le "calqul" économique du consommateur : ce qui s'échange autour d'un chariot. *L'Année sociologique*, 61(1), 71–101.

Cova, B. and Cova, V. (2009). Les figures du nouveau consommateur : une genèse de la gouvernementalité du consommateur. *Recherche et applications en marketing*, 24(3), 81–100.

Denis, J. and Pontille, D. (2010). *Petite sociologie de la signalétique. Les coulisses des panneaux du métro*. Presses des Mines, Paris.

Dichter, E. (1961). *La stratégie du désir. Une philosophie de la vente*. Fayard, Paris.

Dubuisson-Quellier, S. (2003). Confiance et qualité des produits alimentaires : une approche par la sociologie des relations marchandes. *Sociologie du travail*, 45(1), 95–111.

Dubuisson-Quellier, S. (2016). *Gouverner les conduites*. Presses de Sciences Po, Paris.

Dubuisson-Quellier, S. and Neuville, J.-P. (2003). *Juger pour échanger*. Éditions de la MSH/Inra, Paris.

François, P. (2011). *Vie et mort des institutions marchandes*. Presses de Sciences Po, Paris.

Geiger, S., Harrison, D., Kjellberg, H., Mallard, A. (2014). *Concerned Markets: Economic Ordering for Multiple Values*. Edward Elgar Publishing Ltd, Cheltenham.

Goldhaber, M.H. (1997). The attention economy and the Net. *First Monday*, 2(4).

Guichard, L., Dedieu, F., Jeuffroy, M.-H., Meynard, J.-M., Reau, R., Savini, I. (2017). Le plan Écophyto de réduction d'usage des pesticides en France : décryptage d'un échec et raisons d'espérer. *Cahiers Agricultures*, 1–12. doi: 10.1051/cagri/2017004

Hutchins, E. (1993). Learning to navigate. In *Understanding Practice: Perspectives on Activity and Context*, Chaiklin, S. and Lave, J. (eds). Cambridge University Press, Cambridge.

Karpik, L. (1989). L'économie de la qualité. *Revue française de sociologie*, 30(2), 187–210.

Laurent, B. and Mallard, A. (eds) (2020). Introduction labels in economic and political life: Studying labelling in contemporary markets. In *Labelling the Economy*. Palgrave Macmillan, London.

Libaert, T. and Allard-Huver, F. (2014). La communication sur les sujets sensibles au prisme des sciences de l'information et de la communication. *Revue de communication sociale et publique*, 81–100.

Morris, J.W. and Murray, S. (2018). *Appified: Culture in the Age of Apps*. University of Michigan Press, Ann Arbor.

North, D. (1990). *Institutions, Institutional Change and Economic Performance*. Cambridge University Press, Cambridge.

Pahun, J. (2020). L'agriculture face aux politiques alimentaires. Une analyse comparée dans trois régions françaises. PhD Thesis, Université Paris-Est, Paris.

Pierson, P. (2000). Increasing returns, path dependence, and the study of politics. *American Political Science Review*, 94(2), 251–267.

Steiner, P. and Trespeuch, M. (2015). *Marchés contestés : quand le marché rencontre la morale*. Presses Universitaires du Mirail, Toulouse.

Stiglitz, J. (1987). The causes and consequences of the dependence of quality on price. *Journal of Economic Literature*, 25(1), 1–48.

3

Activist Measures and Legal Levers: An Interview with Dominique Masset

This interview was conducted by Nataly Botero, Hélène Ledouble and François Allard-Huver on July 4, 2022, via videoconference.

Dominique Masset is an activist, member of the *Faucheurs Volontaires* collective, initiator and co-chairman of the Campagne Glyphosate and co-chairman of the *Secrets toxiques* campaign. In this interview, he discusses the origins of his activism, the various forms of environmental struggle (legal action, communication, media relations) and his worldview, which drives these struggles.

There are numerous environmental issues that sometimes compete with one another. What led you to take an interest in pesticides in your career as an activist?

It is quite a story, as I am an old activist. I started my activist career at the age of 15 in different movements. In the beginning, they were mainly extreme left-wing movements. I could be criticized later for having been a Maoist-Trotskyist at one point, but it was just a phase in my life. Then, I traveled a lot and, among other things, I came across the problems concerning pesticides, notably through my trips to India, where I witnessed DDT being used without any protection, even though it had already been banned in Western countries. After becoming involved in the anti-nuclear movement, I joined the 36-day fast against the resumption of the EPR

Chapter written by Nataly BOTERO, Hélène LEDOUBLE and François ALLARD-HUVER.

project in 2004. My activism gradually led me to join the "Faucheurs volontaires" (GMO crop reapers)[1].

For the Faucheurs, the fundamentals of their struggles are GMOs, pesticides and the patenting of living organisms. Initially, our work mainly focused on GMOs, but from 2016 to 2017 onward, it turned to pesticides, through the actions we carried out in garden centers. For me, these actions and the ensuing lawsuits were an opportunity to delve deeper into the pesticide issue, in order to raise awareness of the subject. This led to "*Campagne Glyphosate*"[2] and then to "*Secrets toxiques*"[3], a whole line of campaigns which have now produced results and evidence supporting the non-application of the law.

I also did a lot of work on nuclear power, as well as 3G and 4G antennas. On climate issues, I was part of groups fighting for climate justice and environmental struggles. So, I did not limit my actions to pesticides, and I am still involved in many associations on different aspects of environmental issues, but the common thread for the last 20 years has been the Faucheurs.

I am currently very focused on pesticides, because at some point you have to make choices.

When we talk about pesticides, we often talk about our relationship with living things in general. Given that we are living beings, there is the question of our health, but is the primary interest animals, wildlife or human health? Or do you see them as intertwined elements?

Indeed, you cannot tell them apart. We are part of the living world, so as soon as we touch living things, we are directly concerned. Obviously, there are strategic communication problems. To raise awareness, we first need to talk about human health, but we must never forget that we are only part of the living world. Today, unfortunately, we have tangible proof of this in the form of heavy damage on human and animal health, the loss of biodiversity, water, soil and air pollution, etc.

---

1 Since the late 1990s, members of the *Confédération paysanne* (farmers' federation), the Green party and environmental associations have joined forces to reap *roundup ready* transgenic rapeseed. The *Faucheurs Volontaires* is a citizen movement launched in 2003. As the number of volunteers grew, they carried out their first protest in 2004 in the name of the eponymous collective, and drew up a charter. The actions were extended to other crops (pesticide-resistant corn, rapeseed and sunflower, vines and potatoes). Their members are fighting against the artificialization and privatization of living organisms and food crops. See: www.faucheurs-volontaires.fr/.

2 From now on, "CG" in the text.

3 From now on, "ST" in the text.

As you know, we have different methods of action between the Faucheurs, "CG" and "ST", but the objective is always the same. The living, the living and the living.

Can you tell us about how the emergence of the *Campagne Glyphosate* came about?

I started as an activist before the Faucheurs collective even existed. Many of these actions were led by the *Confédération paysanne*. I started protesting in the late 1990s. The *Faucheurs Volontaires* (FV) collective was born in 2003 at the Larzac gathering, and since I was already an activist, I was one of the first to sign up for the creation of this movement.

In 2016–2017, there were major action campaigns in garden centers led by the FV. We painted cans of glyphosate-based pesticides to make them unfit for sale. We painted hundreds of these cans, and there were many actions taken by the Faucheurs in France. Of course, these actions led to court cases, five of them in France. During each of these trials, our lawyers tried to get the courts to question the Court of Justice of the European Union (CJEU) on the validity of the assessment methods and compliance with the precautionary principle listed in the European Constitution. Two courts, Foix and Guingamp, followed the Faucheurs' requests and asked these prejudicial questions.

The Foix trial took place in August 2017. We had to wait until the end of 2019 for the verdict and the ruling of the CJEU. This ruling confirmed what we had been defending: studies must focus on the long-term toxicity of the complete product as marketed, and not just on the molecule declared as active. This ruling of October 1, 2019 now serves as a lever and legal support. Many legal and judicial actions today are based on this fundamental ruling, which provides us with a rereading and confirmation from the CJEU.

For this famous 2017 trial, the 21 defendants, our lawyer and his assistant decided we would attend the trial after having our urine tested for glyphosate. We arrived in court with our urine tests showing that we all had glyphosate in our system. I was the one who had the most and held this shocking record for some time, but there were unfortunately others with more in their system than me.

In view of what happened at the end of 2017 – the renewal of the glyphosate approval saga – we decided to generalize these tests with the Faucheurs from *Ariège* (in France), and to do as many of them as possible to measure the population's levels of glyphosate. The idea was to make people aware of what we would discover through these analyses. Given the results we had obtained with 23 people, which confirmed those already obtained by the association *Générations Futures*, we were convinced that we would probably obtain similar results in the majority of cases. Unfortunately, this was confirmed by the 6,848 analyses we produced.

The CG started from there, at the end of 2017. It took us almost a year to prepare it. It took a long time, because we wanted to test all of the processes we were putting in place so that we could really work on amplifying it, without there being any flaws in our methodology.

How do you ensure that the samples are indisputable? Quite simply, it had to be done in the presence of bailiffs: the toilets had to be visited beforehand, samples were taken in underwear and vials had to be packed and sent to the laboratory by the bailiffs, etc. We also had to finalize the terms of the complaint, the targets, the type of complaint (criminal complaint) and test its admissibility. Of course, our lawyer helped us to finalize it.

We tested the first complaints with a few Faucheurs who had already done their analyses for the trial. A case number arrived a month later, confirming that a preliminary investigation was scheduled.

We carried out many more series of analyses to test how it worked, until we decided to launch the operation nationwide, offering volunteer organizers an educational kit on a USB key, with detailed protocols, documents, tutorials and campaign films. By the end of 2008, two other local committees had been set up by *Faucheurs Volontaires* coordinators, because we initially relied on this network. However, we wanted to broaden the scope, so that it would not be a "Faucheurs" campaign, but citizen action.

There was a boom in 2019: 72 local committees were formed and a large number of tests were started, and we were totally overwhelmed by the success of the operation. We acquired 6,848 tests, with around 5,400 complaints filed.

It was a great success and a very strong focus, with colossal media coverage, because we had chosen to lodge complaints in local courts, with instructions – which were generally respected – to call a press conference and send out a press release. We wanted this to be relayed locally to reach as many people as possible, even to those who would not do their own analysis, so that they would be aware that, in their department, "X" dozen or "X" hundred people had glyphosate in their urine.

Why was glyphosate chosen as a marker for presence in the population? Our choice was not to work solely on glyphosate; the slogan of our action was: "I have pesticides in my urine, do you?". The questions put to the CJEU concerned all types of pesticides. Glyphosate was merely a marker for the fact that the pesticide did not exist in nature before it was massively spread and is therefore a product of chemical and industrial origin. We could have looked for arsenic or AMPA[4], for example, but AMPA may have other sources, and arsenic is obviously naturally present in nature.

The communication error was to call this movement the "*Campagne Glyphoste*". We realize this today, especially since we clearly know that the molecule declared as being "active" is the tree that hides the forest. It is the Trojan horse that allows pesticide manufacturers to hide their highly toxic products behind an active molecule.

Do you think that citizens have the right to propose expertise in scientific controversies? What about the role of scientists and their voice in such matters?

Citizens are not de facto legitimate. To be legitimate, their position must be based on solid information and serious investigation. You cannot claim to be an expert if you just have an interest, a fit of disgust or a fit of anger. We still have to rely on opinions and studies. It is therefore one of the roles of activist groups to collectively explore issues in greater depth, perhaps making them more readable than the scientific studies themselves, which are generally difficult to access. This involves popularizing them, though I do not really like this term, to make them more accessible and to look at them from a different angle to that of a scientist. Of course, scientific expertise can only be challenged on the basis of well-founded, considered opinion. It is not enough to just say: "I am against it, because I am against it"; you have to be able to back it up.

Of course, there can be expert citizen reports, and we are seeing more and more of them, but it is almost always through associations, as part of a collective effort to deepen our understanding. *Générations Futures*, CG and ST, and many others, have produced expert reports. All environmental struggles require expertise to be collective, but it must be based on the scientists' work and fed by controversy.

What led you to choose BioCheck as your laboratory for urinalysis?

First of all, BioCheck was on the market, since *Générations Futures* had called on them. That was obviously the first criterion, but we also looked at other laboratories. Since we were predominantly running a French campaign, we wanted to find French laboratories. However, it was the protocol imposed by the labs that made the decision. We found other labs using chromatography or other methods, but they required freezing and asked for 500 frozen vials so they could start work.

4 AMPA (aminomethylphosphonic acid) is a by-product of glyphosate degradation, but it may have other sources.

This made the process terribly complicated, much more expensive and made it virtually impossible for small local groups to be able to do the sampling themselves. BioCheck allows for simple sampling in a vial that has just been soaked in simmering water for 10 minutes, sent by Chronopost.

We have also been refused by certain laboratories who, when asked the question and the reasons for our request, refused. Why? How? You can think up all sorts of answers, but they refused to take our business. So, to sum up, it is essentially a problem of costs, of processes that were really too complicated with the other laboratories. We do not regret it, because we know that we made the right choice, thanks to comparative analyses carried out with CG scientists, which consisted of "doping" vials and sending them blind to two laboratories, including BioCheck. However, it was only on a small number of samples. These tests were just intended to reassure us at a time when we were subject to numerous attacks regarding the choice of the BioCheck laboratory and had committed a huge number of citizens to this venture. As we had asked CRIIGEN[5] to be an expert witness at the future trial, they wanted to confirm that our analyses were reliable before accepting.

They therefore performed a much deeper study themselves, on their own initiative, on a larger sample and on higher doping levels, in two laboratories, including BioCheck. We now have confirmation that BioCheck is totally reliable. It is better on urine than on water, while the other laboratory is better on water than on urine.

For several years now, legal levers have been increasingly used in activist measures. When did they start to be used and what were the obstacles and advantages?

These legal levers have been used for a long time now. Civil disobedience is a means of resistance that has been around since the 19th century with Thoreau – I think of Gandhi here, the abortion struggles, with the "Manifesto of the 343 Sluts" in 1971 – but it has actually developed a lot in the last few years, mainly on environmental and health issues.

For us Faucheurs, it has been an important part of our fight and our leverage. I think we were one of the first movements to use lawsuits almost systematically. Today, we have probably had over 120 trials to date, which is an enormous number. Appeals, cassation, the European Court of Human Rights. We generally push our trials to the limit to help the law evolve and create jurisprudence, as well as for communication.

---

5 Committee for Independent Research and Information on Genetic Engineering (*Comité de recherche et d'informations indépendantes sur le génie génétique*).

It is used in the same way by other associations, as we saw with "*L'Affaire du siècle*"[6]. It is an opportunity to put the spotlight on a problem, a non-compliance with the law.

The Faucheurs have this distinctive feature: it is by breaking the law that we provoke a trial. We go there as defendants, as accused. Whereas, with many associations such as CG or ST, the opposite principle tends to happen: it is the citizen or association who files the complaint.

Obviously, there are numerous advantages, as I said before, but as with all processes, there are also big disadvantages. Perhaps, the main one is that there is no urgency in legal matters, unfortunately. Trials can take a long time: for example, for the 2017 trial, we were still in the Court of Appeal a few weeks ago in Toulouse. Five years later, this case is still before the Court of Cassation, which means another year at the very least! The same goes for the CJEU, where it took two years after our appeal for the Court to issue its ruling. Each time, we stomp our feet because we know that this is a real emergency – an environmental and health emergency. The process drags on and on, and we have to wait in the antechambers of the courts for things to move forward, with all of the setbacks, all of the backlashes that force us to exhaust every possible recourse. This is the big drawback.

A secondary benefit, however, is that we learn how to master the legal tool. Throughout the time I have been taking part in trials and working on them, I have developed skills in this area. I do not see myself as an expert, but I do see myself as a citizen who is well-informed about the workings of the justice system. And, inversely, we also educate our judges. When we arrive in court as defendants who have made deliberate choices, who have solid arguments, we participate in informing the judicial staff present. We never go to trial with less than four or five high-profile witnesses. That is not an insignificant number, and year after year, it is starting to show. Some judges and court staff have become aware of the problems and are taking a different view of our actions. And this is significant. However, I repeat, it is a long, too long-term of a process. It is incredible that there is still no specific unit within the judicial system to deal with environmental issues. There are public health divisions in Paris and Marseille, but regretfully there are no legal divisions in France specializing in environmental problems and the way in which they are handled. We often realize, through court cases, that there are courts that are very far from understanding the problems, and very far from having even scratched the surface of the issue.

6 Campaign against the French state for their lack of action regarding climate change (see: https://laffairedusiecle.net/qui-sommes-nous/).

Farmers despise the fact that their production needs are not being considered, and that they do not have enough alternatives to deal with the ban on certain products (or active substances) that are deemed to be harmful. How would you respond?

Yes, let us talk about alternatives, as there are quite a number of them. After all, around 80% of the world's farmers do not use these chemicals. Our parents and grandparents also did things differently. It has only been since the 1940s and 1950s that we have really seen the development of agrochemicals. Before that, different practices existed and worked. They have been abandoned, and I even think that there is a major loss of knowledge today on the part of farmers, a loss relating to the nature of soils and ecosystems (which plant grows in which environment? What is it predestined for in the context of agricultural production? etc.). There is a real lack of territorial knowledge. I think that has all been more or less lost with the generalization of very large areas, where different types of land are mixed together and should not be growing the same crops. In the village where I lived for a long time, there was a great deal of fragmentation: on the one side, there were potatoes, on the other side, wheat or corn to feed the chickens, and in each place, there was very different work depending on the soil, the slope, the exposure or the natural drainage. That is the first point: alternatives do exist.

The second point is that farmers have, for decades, been accustomed to, initiated and sometimes very much influenced using chemistry as a crutch or support. Indeed, it is difficult for them to move toward the alternatives that exist without real training and support. The question is: how can we get these farmers who have been using chemicals for years to switch to something else? We are talking about transition. However, this transition cannot take place without a strong political decision. As we have seen with the Ecophyto plan, if there is no strong obligation, there is failure, because there is no obligation for farmers, for users of these products, to do things differently: the injunction "you do it if you can" clearly does not work.

This money would have been better spent on agricultural colleges, technicians at the French Chambers of Agriculture, and all of the people who are supposed to give farmers relevant advice. There is a real job to be done here, with no more dithering on the restrictive side. Pesticides must be banned, and assistance in the transition must be implemented, but they first need to be banned. Not a transition and then a ban, because that does not work. The constraint has to be there, with a clearly announced date. For example: "you have three or four years to change your methods, with support for human resources, advice, technical training and financial resources, but once these three or four years have passed, pesticides are over and done with".

To achieve this, we need to think and work hard on current farming methods, such as abandoning monocultures and using very short wheat/sunflower rotations. Many farms are disappearing and are often attributed to expansion rather than installation. This is another very serious political mistake. Today, we continue to give land to expand existing farms, when we should be giving it to create new farms where the surface level allows for agroecological methods, which is obviously almost impossible when working on 300 hectares of cereals, or at the very least extremely complicated. So, it really is time to make a 180 degree turn to really change practices and work in all these areas.

We also need to take stock of local production, and aim for food self-sufficiency. We need to stop having regions that grow too much wheat and others with too many cows. We need to diversify crops and production between livestock and crops. This provides organic matter. I am not a farmer; I have only been a professional beekeeper in my life, but there are some obvious points. And there is experience, and therefore facts, with farmers in France, Europe and all over the world, who work without chemical inputs. All we need is real political will and the means to match.

Certain alternatives to pesticides (known as biocontrol products), such as sulfur and copper, have a potentially negative impact (on health, the environment and, in the case of copper, in the neighborhood through odors). What do you think of their use in place of conventional pesticides?

Bordeaux mixture and sulfur are used as fungicides to treat vines, apple trees and, more generally, plants that are susceptible to fungal attacks. The use of these products is a real problem. To start with, there are ways to reduce the consumption of these products, particularly copper. There is a very interesting INRAE study on the subject, published in 2018[7], which shows that it is possible to obtain the same results with the same number of sprays, but at half the dosage. I would add that the particularity of these products is that they are used preventively, with all of the shortcomings of sometimes being useless, but without the possibility of knowing what would have happened if they had not been used.

In fact, this is one of the attacks made by non-bios against bios, in the specifications in which copper and sulfur are authorized. We can tell them that it is not a synthetic chemical mixture; it is generally one or two molecules. Bordeaux mixture is lime and copper. It is not a cocktail of chemical molecules added on top of each other (it is nothing like what you would find in a chemical pesticide): it is natural minerals. In that

7 See: www.inrae.fr/actualites/biodiversite-services-rendus-nature-que-sait-limpact-pesticides [Accessed January 31, 2023].

respect, it is still a lesser evil. There are successful alternatives too, but they are mainly effective on annual plantings. For established vines and fruit trees, it is much more complicated: prophylaxis through proper management of waste from previous years, plant stimulants (Plant Resistance Inducers) and varietal mixes. It would be interesting to further study these subjects, to see how we can do without these added products. Here, as elsewhere, we need to completely revisit our farming methods and move toward agroecology.

I just wanted to say a word about farmers, and that is that they are not our adversaries and even less so our enemies. They have very big problems; just look at the number of suicides and the number of bankruptcies, which continue to rise.

It takes a great deal of courage to face up to, on a daily basis, the relational problems that farmers can have with their predecessors or parents when they change course, or with other farmers who feel scorned by what they interpret as a challenge to their working methods.

This is precisely where a political decision can alleviate such problems. If everyone is forced to change their farming methods, we will not point the finger at someone who is going to be ostracized from the others, just because they have done something different. It is important to understand how difficult it is today for farmers, especially large-scale farmers, to change their practices, with very strong unions and widespread practice. Forgive me for digressing, but it is important not to pick the wrong target.

Several actions were covered by the media, notably when activists painted glyphosate cans in garden centers. What can you say about these actions? Do you think they are useful (or even convincing) for citizens? Is it to draw attention to the potentially toxic products sold in garden centers (and often packaged in green)? Or is there another objective?

It all depends on the type of action. If we are talking about the glyphosate cans in the garden centers, the initial aim was to shine a spotlight on an issue. This is what activist whistle-blowers, the *Faucheurs Volontaires* and others (Extinction Rebellion, *Les Soulèvements de la Terre*, etc.) do. These are powerful actions, and the aim is to publicize them and hopefully raise awareness of the problem among citizens in a general way, as well as users, professionals and victims alike. The lawsuits that follow are another means of action: there is the action itself, which tries to raise awareness, and the lawsuits that follow, which are a way of highlighting the problem in another way.

Strong nonviolent action can only be symbolic. When we reap a few hectares of GMO sunflowers out of the 200,000 hectares cultivated in France, it is obviously symbolic. We need to use this symbolic action to turn it into a communication tool and a means of spreading awareness. These actions, if carried out at night, masked and unacknowledged, have little meaning or impact. That is why we act openly, providing the police with a list of participants. The *Faucheurs Volontaires* take responsibility for their actions individually, while asserting that they have been decided and carried out collectively.

There are also legal actions, such as the CG. Citizens file complaints against citizens, not against an organization. It is a complaint against the people in charge of these organizations, and that is practically unique. We have filed a complaint against people we have not named, but whose functions we have. The aim is not to lodge a complaint against an organization, because when Monsanto became Bayer, any prior complaint would have been dropped.

It was also intended to bring those who make decisions for us out of anonymity. It is extremely important that they become the clear target of a legal procedure, whereby they are held personally responsible for the acts they have committed. This is fundamental for CG: a complaint by a group of individuals against a group of individuals.

Then there is ST, a complaint by associations against national or European structures for failure to apply the law. ST has lodged a criminal complaint against X, and it will then be up to the Paris public prosecutor's office to find out who is responsible. However, the main focus of CG's and ST's actions is to ensure compliance with European and French regulations on pesticide assessment and approval methods. ST is working to ensure compliance with the law. We have gathered, filmed and recorded evidence that the law is not being respected, either by the European Commission and EFSA, or by the French government and ANSES.

There are other potential targets, but those used in these three types of actions are different, concordant and complementary. CG relies on the action of the Faucheurs through the CJEU's ruling, and ST can rely on CG's result to get illustrations of what it does. ST was initiated by *Générations Futures*, *Nature et Progrès* and CG, and today has over 60 member associations and local groups, from large NGOs to small local associations.

Getting back to legal and communication strategies; until now, complaints were lodged directly by lawyers with the Paris public prosecutor's office. However, from now on, in several regions, complaints will be lodged by local associations in their local courts. For the same reasons as for CG, this is an opportunity to hold a press conference and write press articles. Each filing serves to communicate ST findings and actions, and the illegality of the valuation principles.

In terms of campaigns, what are the methods of action, the images and the speeches that succeed in mobilizing the greatest number of people? What are the powerful symbols, as the media are fond of this type of action? What becomes audible and can be picked up by the media?

I am going to talk about the *Faucheurs Volontaires* (FV) again, since I am familiar with this example, even though I often take part in other types of action led by other groups. The targets of the FV are, of course, GMOs, as well as pesticides and the patenting of living organisms. These are collective actions, carried out with thoughtful, widely debated communication. We choose our targets. Generally speaking, we begin by providing information and sounding the alarm: leaflets, press articles, conferences, petitions, meetings with MPs, ministers, etc. When all of this work fails to produce results, we move on to acts of civil disobedience.

As I said earlier, these nonviolent actions are mainly symbolic. Take, for example, the pesticide cans: often, their labels have been cleaned and the cans put back on sale. This example of the Faucheurs' action in garden centers is a concrete example of the shockwave that can be caused by a small action of 20 people in a small garden center in a small county, and which, in the end, questions the whole of Europe and today serves us as legal leverage.

We raided BASF premises in Lyon and discovered pesticides that were banned in France and should no longer exist in France, or be exported. We did an ad on the subject and communicated: "Who is illegal? BASF or us?".

Apart from glyphosate, what are the other most symbolic products or molecules that the general public is calling for to be regulated or banned?

Many of us now find it increasingly difficult to talk about a molecule. I think we must urgently change the way we approach the issue and talk about it. We were recently received by the European Parliament, and this meeting was extremely useful to us. We need to stop talking about active molecules, and talk about the complete product as marketed. We need to talk about the product, because the active molecule is really a lure that turns against us: how can we rebel against the use of acetic acid or pelargonic acid as a pesticide? If we analyze the whole can, we know that it contains all of the toxins and poisons found in all chemical pesticides. We know that the active molecule is a way of passing off a product that has a pesticidal effect but whose toxicity is acceptable in terms of current standards, while concealing the real toxicity of the complete product. The controversy between the study carried out by the Institute of Cancer Research (IARC)[8] and EFSA[9] is that one studied glyphosate and the other studied Roundup. The IARC conducted a study on the finished product, and indeed, the toxicity rate is very different from that of an active molecule.

So, I find it hard to answer this question, especially given that, apart from glyphosate, chlordecone, neonicotinoids and a few others, there are not many molecules that get media coverage, so for the general public, pesticide equals glyphosate. It should be noted that surveys have shown that a large majority of French people want pesticides to be banned.

And what about neonicotinoids? Thanks to questions about beetroots this is becoming increasingly visible, even though we have been using them for 30 years and no one had ever heard of them. Is it this whole political effect of prohibition, reauthorization and derogation that is making it visible?

The government itself has brought neonicotinoids to light by banning them and granting derogations, hence the outcry. The lobbies did their bit, led by the FNSEA[10], who blocked the roads with their big farming machinery, which they know how to do. Lobbying is very influential, and we have a lot to worry about in terms of glyphosate approval being renewed.

We all know that the climate issue has become central to environmental action. So what role does the pesticide issue currently play in society?

It is not peripheral. If all of these actions against pesticides succeed, they will lead to a different type of agriculture, which is one of the answers to the climate problem. We want to implement agroecology, a natural form of agriculture that will emit much less and capture many more greenhouse gases, maintain soil moisture, reduce flooding and stop killing the farmer's work tool: the soil. It is not just about agriculture, but it is an important aspect.

---

8 The International Agency for Research on Cancer (IARC) is an agency forming part of the World Health Organization (see: https://www.iarc.who.int/).
9 European Food Safety Authority (see: https://www.efsa.europa.eu/en).
10 The French national farmers' union (see: https://www.fnsea.fr/).

However, we realize from ST that it is hard to get people hooked. It was much easier with the CG action, which proposed concrete action. ST is the result of two years' work, and it is legal procedure. It is based on legal texts that we have dissected, and they are not easy to deal with. It is true that it does not attract the public or the media. The latter were very keen on the glyphosate actions. However, telling them, "you know, in the assessment methods, there's such and such a flaw, such and such a practice that does not work" does not really interest them.

It is quite complicated to raise public awareness of pesticides. Even if a survey shows that 80% of French people would like to be without pesticides, this issue is not the focal point. It is really just one element in a web of problems that need to be resolved and tackled globally.

When we tackle pesticides, we are dealing with the whole oil industry, the whole issue of international trade, globalization and product transport, and food self-sufficiency. There are many other points on which we need to work, and we are all trying to do so at our own level.

If we manage to enforce the law on pesticides, we will eliminate 95% of them. If we calculate the true long-term toxicity of these products, they are virtually all unmarketable, being extremely dangerous and toxic. There is a real need for scientific and industrial research to create safe tools. ST has made a film that starts with alternatives, with agroecology. We have made a lot of progress since the film came out, but as soon as we discover one flaw, others appear. ST is currently working with other associations to create a pesticide map, trying to identify all of the problems and the actors working around this issue. The idea is to produce a summary to provide a tool for MPs, decision-makers, the media and anyone else who wants to have as much information as possible at their fingertips. For example, we recently came across a study on PPE (personal protective equipment), which shows that it is ineffective, and that it is even more dangerous because users, feeling protected, take far fewer precautions than if they were not wearing it. Those who wear it have more pesticides on their skin than those who do not.

We are trying to globalize the problem. One example: in a province in India, they are in the process of defining a chemical-free agriculture, with the aim of achieving food self-sufficiency. Changing the type of agriculture is a systemic approach. If we manage to ban 90% or 95% of pesticides, many things will change for living beings and society in general.

Have you seen any changes in the way the issue has been handled by the media, say over the past 10 years or so? And how would you describe your relations with the media?

Yes, there are changes, but they are seasonal or mainstream changes: one day, there is an ad on glyphosate; another day it is on something else, and they do not talk about pesticides at all. These are seasons when everyone is outbidding one another, focusing on an issue or an event. Most media are event-driven. For activists, it is all about creating events to attract the media: they need images, buzz and to get things moving.

When it comes to in-depth work, it is much more complicated. It is a bit like what I was saying about the ST campaign: it is much harder to get them to look into it, because there are not many investigative journalists on the subject, just as there are not many courts on the subject. We would need a Marie-Monique Robin in every media outlet to really do a serious investigation.

I have my doubts and concerns about the way in which the media are handling this issue. Our relations with the media vary greatly. You can have a press release that falls into complete media silence, a press conference at which you are left with two or three friends and the local media taking part. And then at another moment, 30 or 40 media outlets are present. So, why? Probably because there is not too much else to get your teeth into, because you are doing an event and it fills up the media everywhere, and then it dies down again.

There are not enough genuinely independent media outlets that get to the heart of the issues, and are not just there to report the news and create a buzz. Too many media outlets have little or no counterweight. They used to oppose current policies. We hope that the French National Assembly and the European Parliament will be able to play this role to some extent.

To conclude, we are going to leave the media sphere for those who decide on European regulations. There will be debates on the reauthorization of glyphosate in December 2022. Do you think legislators are sufficiently informed to act?

This is really the crux of the matter: there is a real need for legislators and decision-makers to be informed. Some of them are, and they know what they are doing; they are responsible for their choices. However, there is also a real lack of knowledge, both among the courts and among European politicians. For almost a year and a half now, we have been having one meeting a week with national and European MPs, lobbying them hard, and we realize that they are increasingly aware of the reality of the problem. The reality is that the finished product is not really assessed as it should be.

We are going to lodge an appeal with the *Conseil d' État* (French Council of State), along with other MPs and associations from the ST coalition. Some MPs have really become aware. We went to the European Parliament two weeks ago for a conference and there were around 50 participants, including parliamentary secretaries and members of parliament.

Nevertheless, there are major shortcomings in the understanding of these issues, and this is understandable. A parliamentarian should be competent in a thousand different fields, and this is totally impossible. The lobbying work we do clearly counteracts the lobbying on the other side, but we do not have the same means, and fortunately, not the same methods.

ST has submitted a petition to the European Parliament: any citizen or association can question the Parliament if they consider that one of the European bodies is not respecting the law. In addition, we will be launching actions for the termination of two or three products that will be renewed in the coming months. We are working on an action for failure to act, which will be lodged as soon as we have made sufficient progress in our lobbying work to hope that Parliament will take up the issue.

An example of the misinformation that certain state bodies are capable of producing: we have, for example, a study showing that there are many highly toxic products in biocontrol products based on acetic, pelargonic or caprylic acid, elements that have not been declared on the label[11]. ANSES commissioned a second opinion from the French Commission on Competition, Consumption and Fraud (DGCCRF)[12]. With great difficulty, we were able to obtain this "second opinion". The report does not specify the method used, the molecules researched are not the same, and lastly, the level of quantification is five to ten times higher than that used by Professor Séralini's generic.

There is a blatant lack of transparency, scientific rigor and ongoing control. French National and European food safety agencies use studies produced by manufacturers on the "active" molecule declared by the petitioner. They rely on data from the Registration, Evaluation and Authorization of Chemicals (REACH)[13], data which is often incomplete and all too often nonexistent for the few declared "co-formulants".

11 See: https://www.sciencedirect.com/science/article/pii/S0278691520306608.

12 Original French: *Direction générale de la concurrence, de la consommation et de la répression des fraudes* (DGCCRF).

13 Data available on the following website: www.prc.cnrs.fr/reach/fr/data_requirements.html.

Based on this incomplete data, they define the toxicity of so-called "representative" formulations, using computer modeling that has not been disseminated or calibrated by comparative experimental study. In this respect, I think we can call these methods aberrations.

This is an urgent situation: people are falling ill every day, biodiversity is collapsing and the climate is going wild. Despite the obvious, we are obliged to explain the consequences of using these poisons again and again.

4

The Globalization of Regulatory Science on Pesticides: History and Effects on European Law

4.1. Introduction

This chapter offers a legal and historical perspective on international approaches to the use of pesticides. By answering the questions concerning the tools and ideas which have presided over the constitution of regulatory science on pesticides, including the effects within the European Union, we show that regulatory science is globalized and, as a result, is moving towards European law while concealing certain harmful effects.

From a methodological point of view, the corpus of documents used, whether or not they have a normative purpose, was formed thanks to their online publication. The period studied extends from the late 1960s to the present day. There is a twofold approach. Firstly, it is based on an analysis at both an international and regional level of the formal sources of law and the standards of soft law, which are generic expressions for legally nonbinding tools, some of which nonetheless have real normative power. It also draws on disciplines other than law, for two reasons. The first is the chemical nature of pesticides, whose health and environmental effects call on a number of disciplines from the so-called hard sciences. The case law of the Court of Justice of the European Union (CJEU) on pesticides bears witness, both in the parties' arguments and in the judges' reasoning, to the complex terms of the dialogue between law and these various sciences. This interdisciplinary approach is essential for lawyers wishing to understand, explain and perhaps criticize the legal framework. The second reason, which brings us to the edges of sociology, political science and

Chapter written by Annie MARTIN.

the history of science, is the fact that nongovernmental organizations (NGOs), the press, scientists and public bodies are regularly highlighting (Jouzel 2019) and denouncing a shift between the regulations that make the marketing of pesticides conditional on the production of science proving that this chemical object has no unacceptable effects on the environment and health, and another science, which would be no less consensual[1] and would prove that authorized pesticides have harmful effects.

Since 2009, environmental scientists have been arguing that chemical pollution, which interacts with biodiversity and climate change, is one of the nine planetary boundaries that human activity must not transgress, if we are to avoid unacceptable global environmental change (Rockström et al. 2009). Continuing this work, other scientists asserted in 2022 that no regulatory assessment can include all of the possible impacts of the 350,000 chemical products[2] on the market, in other words, that their production exceeds global assessment and monitoring capacity, and that this constitutes a transgression that affects the Earth system's capacity for self-regulation. This recent study concludes that increasing production is incompatible with maintaining humanity in a safe operating space (Persson et al. 2022). These scientific publications are echoed at the institutional level. The Organisation for Economic Cooperation and Development (OECD), a major player in the globalization of pesticide regulatory science, admits that there is insufficient risk assessment for 20,000–100,000 approved chemical products (OECD 2015, p. 11). The *Office parlementaire d'évaluation des choix scientifiques et technologiques* (French Parliamentary Office for the Evaluation of Scientific and Technological Choices) states that "pesticides present a particularly significant threat to insects due to [...] inadequate risk assessment regulations" at both the European and national level (OPECST 2021, p. 2). The *Commission nationale de la déontologie et des alertes en santé publique et environnement* (French National Commission on Ethics and Alerts in Public Health and the Environment), which commissioned experts to reflect on improving "the articulation between 'regulatory science' and 'academic science'" in the consideration of chemical risks, reached the same conclusion (Bonvallot et al. 2021, pp. 3 and 24)[3]. It was along these lines that, in January 2022, five associations[4] brought action against the French government for negligence in

1 The supplementary brief to the petition lodged by several associations against the French state with the Paris Administrative Court on January 10, 2022, refers to "a scientific consensus" that "agrochemical pollution due to the use of plant protection products is one of the main factors in the widespread decline in biodiversity".

2 The term *chemical products* is used in the broad sense used in the study, including plant protection products, biocides, cosmetics, etc.

3 The report uses a family of SDHi fungicides, glyphosate and neonicotinoids as examples.

4 Notre affaire à tous, POLLINIS, Biodiversité sous nos pieds, l'Association nationale pour la protection des eaux et rivières Truite-Ombre-Saumon and l'Association pour la protection des animaux sauvages et du patrimoine naturel.

the assessment and authorization procedures for plant protection products (PPPs). This action, called "Justice pour le vivant"[5], points, for example, to the failure to consider several aspects in the assessment of indirect effects, notably trophic interactions[6] and cumulative or cocktail effects, in other words, the interaction between the substances contained in a single complex product, on the one hand, and the multiple substances and compounds present in the environment, on the other.

These various forms of public and often collective mobilization have one thing in common: they highlight the inadequacy of regulatory science, an expression whose use is appropriate in the context of this reflection, even though it is foreign to French-speaking academic legal discourse. Formalized in the early 1990s, regulatory science is understood as a "set of scientific assessment activities that participate in taking legal measures aimed at framing industrial activities and products" and whose criteria and procedures "are formalized in regulatory texts, guidelines" (Demortain and Borraz 2015, p. 279). In concrete terms, these rules and standards are, for the most part, technical in nature, determining the scientific protocols that make it possible, for example, to identify the effects of endocrine disruption[7]. They deal with scientific issues such as the animal species that can be used for testing. The implementation of these standards results in the production of regulatory knowledge on the effects of chemical substances. Regulatory science is therefore at the heart of expert decision-making, and we can observe the recent emergence of the expression in the discourse of European institutions[8] such as the Council (Council of the European Union 2021, pp. 27 and 31), the Parliament (European Parliament and Council 2019, p. 60) and the Commission (European Commission 2020a, p. 17). Its use reflects the coexistence of two sciences: the one enshrined in the rules for the pre-market assessment of pesticides, which legitimizes both the knowledge produced and the trade in these products, and the one conducted outside any normative perspective. In social science research, however, regulatory science is criticized for the influence that industrialists exert on its content through various tools such as lobbying, links and conflicts of interest, and revolving doors (Demortain 2017). The risk of industrial influence on the fight against the harmful effects of pesticides can be seen in practice, since the Food and Agriculture Organization of the United Nations announced its collaboration with the pesticide industry trade association CropLife International. The event has prompted reactions from scientists and NGOs (Gérard 2020), who condemn a conflict of interest with the UN's mission and mandate to protect biodiversity, support the public good, and respect, protect and fulfill human rights. In the same vein, European law bears witness to the pressure exerted by interest representatives on regulatory

5 "Justice for the living". See: www.justicepourlevivant.org/ [Accessed January 19, 2023].
6 All of the interactions between living beings in an ecosystem.
7 The term emerged in 1991 and refers to the disruption of the hormonal system, whether human or animal, by chemical substances and products.
8 There are only a few search results for the term *regulatory science* on the European Union's Eurlex site, but they start in 2013 in the drug sector.

science. For example, the European regulation concerning the placing of PPPs on the market (European Parliament and Council 2009a, hereinafter the PPP Regulation[9]) required the Commission to present scientific criteria for determining endocrine-disrupting properties by December 2013 at the latest. As substances with endocrine-disrupting properties cannot be used in pesticides, industry lobbied so hard that the Commission failed to meet the deadline and was brought before the European General Court (EGC), which – exceptionally – ruled against it for failure to act. To justify its delay, the Commission lightly invoked "criticisms" of the scientific criteria it had proposed in terms of their impact on the internal market (EGC 2015, paragraph 69). On the other hand, it was more audacious in referring to "interference by external parties" and "undue pressure" from representatives of interests (EGC 2016, paragraph 27) to oppose the communication of all documents relating to the draft regulations to an NGO. As the EGC points out, the Commission preferred to confine itself to "general, vague and imprecise indications" (EGC 2016, paragraph 32), and it was outside the jurisdiction of the courts that industrial pressure was documented (Horel 2015). Similarly, the European Ombudsman has criticized the Commission for not requiring a declaration of interest from academic experts whose research is cofinanced by the chemical industry, when they take part in training workshops to prepare a method for assessing the environmental risks of pesticides (European Ombudsman 2021).

With these clarifications in mind, it is now time to define pesticides in European law. The term, in use since the late 1960s, was not defined until 1978 in a sense that was close to its Latin etymology, in other words, as mixtures intended alternatively to "destroy" "organisms harmful to plants", "undesired plants", "parts of plants", "promote [...] plant production" and "preserve plant products" (Council of the European Union 1978a, Article 2). In the same year, the term "pesticide" coexisted with the term "plant protection product", which was used to denote similar effects (Council of the European Union 1978b, Article 2) with a preference to mean that these products aim to "protect plants [...] against [...] harmful organisms" (Council of the European Union 1991, Article 2; European Parliament and Council 2009a, Article 2.a). In 2009, the term *pesticide* became generic, with European law (European Parliament and Council 2009b, Article 3) expressly stating that pesticides cover two categories of products governed by different texts: PPPs for agricultural use and biocides for other uses, the main ones being disinfection of people, animals and things (water, surfaces, materials, etc.), antimicrobial protection and pest control[10]. The PPPs covered in this chapter are defined as "products, [...] consisting of or containing [...] active substances, safeners or synergists [...]" (European

9 Current text.

10 The European Chemicals Agency (ECHA) distinguishes 22 types of biocides in four main groups. See: www.echa.europa.eu/fr/regulations/biocidal-products-regulation/product-types [Accessed November 8, 2022].

Parliament and Council 2009a, Article 2). A PPP is therefore a complex product, a mixture generally composed of several chemical objects, which are either individual substances or mixtures of several substances. Roundup, for example, is a PPP composed of an active substance, glyphosate, and other substances or mixtures of substances.

In simple terms, PPP Regulation makes market access for PPPs subject to a two-stage procedure. Active substances, safeners and synergists are subject to a European approval procedure carried out by Rapporteur Member States, the European Food Safety Authority (EFSA) and the Commission, which grants or withholds approval, and may or may not renew it. The PPP, or finished product, which may only contain active substances, PPPs and synergists[11] approved by the Commission, is subject to a national but harmonized marketing authorization procedure. In the light of "current scientific and technical knowledge" (Article 4.1 and Article 29.1.e), these two levels consist of an assessment to ensure that PPP residues have no harmful effect on human health and no unacceptable effect on the environment (Article 4.2), and that the PPP is sufficiently effective, has no immediate or delayed harmful effects on human health and has no unacceptable effects on plants or the environment (Article 4.3).

This expert system and the current state of scientific and technical knowledge targeted by the PPP Regulation are specifically influenced by one international organization (IO) in particular, the OECD, which globalizes the regulatory science it develops. In the general field of the environment, with which chemical safety is linked at the OECD, the latter has adopted 97 tools that illustrate its normative power, or at least a capacity to influence or persuade (SFDI 2013). The polluter-pays economic principle formalized by the OECD, which is now incorporated into international environmental law, is a striking example of this power and of the translation of an economic principle into the legal system at international and national levels. The OECD has been a pioneer in formulating and integrating an economic aspect into environmental policies and, in its words, in "the definition of effective and efficient environmental policies [...]" (OECD 2011a, p. 9). Since the 1970s, acting as a lever to propose a harmonized model, the OECD has globalized ideas and tools containing scientific methods for producing knowledge on the health and environmental effects of chemical products used in PPPs. The dissemination of these methods to member states and other IOs leads to the harmonization of knowledge. It is surprising that the OECD has taken on the task of drawing up

11 A PPP may also contain co-formulants as defined in Article 2.3.c of the PPP Regulation, provided they are not on the list of prohibited co-formulants. However, co-formulants are not subject to the approval procedure established by this regulation. They are solely governed by the REACH regulation (European Parliament and Council 2006, Article 14) which, unlike the PPP Regulation, only requires the production of certain knowledge for substances produced in quantities exceeding 10 tons.

standards in this field. It is not a scientific organization, and its primary objective is not to protect health and the environment, but to promote economic growth. To this end, it has sought to build trust in knowledge about the effects of chemical products, thereby helping to facilitate the flow of trade in these products. To do this, however, it had to build trust in the way knowledge is produced. This aspect is at the heart of the rules and standards we will examine in section 4.2, before looking at their effects on European law in section 4.3.

4.2. Chemical safety ideas and tools promoted worldwide by the OECD

According to the first article of its founding Convention, the OECD, which groups together 38 countries committed to market economy principles, has the objective of promoting policies particularly designed "to achieve the highest sustainable economic growth [...], and thus to contribute to the development of the world economy" (OECD 1960). In the chemical sector, the promotion of world trade has underpinned the OECD's work from the outset. According to the organization, the tools it has adopted have contributed to the expansion[12] of the global chemical industry, which has become the second largest industry in the world (UNEP 2019, p. 24). The rapid growth of the chemical market has benefited OECD member countries, where 83% of world production was concentrated when it began publishing its work on chemical trade in 1970 (OECD 2011b, p. 4)[13].

4.2.1. *Ideas promoted by the OECD in the chemical sector*

Collective awareness of the environmental and health hazards posed by chemical products dates back to the publication of Silent Spring (Carson 1962). At the time, the Council of Europe was a pioneer in environmental matters (Meyer 2017, p. 7), and as early as 1968, adopted various texts for its protection, including in the chemical sector. At the same time, the increase in product safety regulations in the US (Jones and Benrubi 2013, p. 802) threatened to create trade barriers in the chemical sector. Concerned about the economic impact of emerging environmental policies, and in particular about the creation of non-tariff barriers to trade that divergent national laws would foster (OECD 1977a), the OECD quickly responded by creating the Committee on the Environment in 1970 (now called the Environment Policy Committee). From the outset, the Secretary General's speech emphasized the cost of pollution control programs for companies, which had measurable consequences on their profitability and economic performance. He advocated the

12 Its value increased sevenfold between 1978 and 2008, from $520 billion to $3,697 billion (OECD 2010, p. 12).

13 Chemical production in OECD countries still accounts for almost 60% of the world total (OECD 2019, p. 13).

introduction of measures that did not have a negative impact on trade and economic growth (Meyer 2017, p. 2). Two years after the creation of the United Nations Environment Program (UNEP) and the US ban on DDT, this committee, which worked with the Chemicals Committee under the aegis of the OECD's Environment Directorate, developed (OECD 1974) the two ideas pursued by the tools that are currently in effect.

The first idea, which was the need to assess the health and environmental effects of chemicals before they are marketed, emerged outside the OECD, at the United Nations Conference on the Human Environment in Stockholm, in 1972[14]. However, this idea became secondary to another relating to the mutual acceptance of data, according to which each OECD member state must trust the results of the pre-market assessment of chemical substances carried out by any other member country. This idea has an economic rationale.

Indeed, the OECD has chosen an economic direction, citing the 1972 Guiding Principles concerning International Economic Aspects of Environmental Policies in the first citation of the text adopted in 1974. It was in this guiding principle that the OECD first enunciated the polluter-pays economic principle, designed in particular to maintain the environment in an "acceptable state" (OECD 1972, Appendix, A.a. points 3 and 4). At the time, the OECD stated that, "in many circumstances [...] the reduction of pollution beyond a certain level will not be practical or even necessary in view of the costs involved". From this economic perspective, the OECD also stated that "measures taken to protect the environment should be framed [...] to avoid the creation of non-tariff barriers to trade". In the chemical sector, the OECD recommended that the governments of member countries consider "in particular" the "financial resources" required for pre-assessment and select "those chemicals that require a full-scale assessment" (OECD 1974).

The idea of mutual acceptance of data is also explained by the principle of efficient use of economic resources enshrined in Article 2.a of the OECD Convention. Assessing the toxicity of chemicals requires time, as well as technical and financial resources, which are all the more important given that the OECD's objective was the growth of this market. The efficient use of these resources justified the introduction of the system of trust between states, since it avoids the need for governments and companies to incur the expenses required by the evaluation, when it has already been carried out by an OECD member state.

The consequence of this economic reasoning was endorsed in 1977 in a recommendation (OECD 1977a) aimed at preparing a hard law text. While the

14 The Conference agreed on the need to "raise awareness and give advance warning of the harmful effects of man-made pollutants on human health and well-being" (Recommendation 74).

Council recognized the desirability of evaluating all chemical products, it chose, in view of the resources available, to limit control to new chemical substances and to certain existing substances, with the exception of products made from these substances. This may well be the point of origin of the lack of knowledge about the cocktail effects of chemicals that is being denounced today (Rockström et al. 2009; UNEP 2019, p. 163; OPECST 2021, p. 3). The OECD itself points out in its latest Environmental Outlook that, in OECD member countries, "the health impacts of chemicals [...] in the environment – and in particular effects from combined exposure to mixtures of chemicals – is still limited" (OECD 2012, p. 26).

4.2.2. *Tools developed by the OECD in the chemical sector*

Still in effect today, the Council Decision on Mutual Acceptance of Data in the Assessment of Chemicals (hereinafter MAD) was adopted in 1981 (OECD 1981). The MAD is a hard law tool with a legal scope that is equivalent to that of an international treaty. In the typology of acts provided for by the OECD Convention, a decision is, in principle, adopted by common agreement by all members and is binding, subject to compliance with the constitutional procedure in effect in each country (OECD 1960, Article 6.1, Article 5a and Article 6.3). The choice of this tool is all the more significant given that the OECD, whose action is based on persuading members to pursue certain types of policy, favors nonbinding measures[15].

The MAD is divided into two very short parts and two appendices. The body of the decision contains certain omissions. It does not transform the idea of assessing the health and environmental effects of chemicals before they are marketed into a rule of substantive law. This idea is still conveyed by soft law, namely the 1974 Recommendation (OECD 1974), to which the MAD decision refers. More significantly, the MAD mentions virtually no minimum or systematic obligation to assess chemical substances and does not require the assessment of new or existing substances. On this point, the OECD subsequently adopted a binding decision, requiring member states to implement or strengthen national programs for the systematic examination of existing chemicals (OECD 1987). The MAD does not distinguish between products and substances, the former being generally considered a combination of the latter. Other IOs and individual states are therefore free to introduce rules on these issues. Lastly, the MAD does not say whether it is up to governments or industry to provide evidence of the effects of chemicals. We have to look at the preparatory work of the Environment Committee to find out that it is up to the manufacturer to carry out the initial assessment of a substance (OECD 1977b).

---

15 In the chemical sector, 20 OECD texts are in effect, including 11 Recommendations, eight Decisions or Decisions–Recommendations, and one Declaration.

In the first part, the MAD expressly lays down the principle of sharing test data as a legally binding rule:

> Data generated in the testing of chemicals in an OECD Member country in accordance with OECD Test Guidelines and OECD Principles of Good Laboratory Practice shall be accepted in other Member countries for the purpose of assessment and other uses relating to the protection of man and the environment.

To ensure that the obligation to accept data is effective, the MAD makes the production of such data subject to two conditions: testing must be carried out in accordance with what the OECD calls "test guidelines" and "principles of good laboratory practice" (GLP). In essence, these guidelines and GLP constitute OECD regulatory science and the key to mutual trust between states, a prerequisite for growth in the chemical product trade.

The second part of the MAD does not contain any obligations, but rather a recommendation inviting states to apply the guidelines and GLP contained in the two appendices. The term "recommendation" suggests that the guidelines and GLP are soft law, whereas they are contained in a legally binding decision and form the cornerstone of the system. In practical terms, Appendix I of the decision lists five series of guidelines adopted or revised since 1981[16]. For example, guideline 234 for the Fish Sexual Development Test, which concerns endocrine disruption, indicates which fish species are selected for testing, the reasons for these choices and which indicators, including the evolution of the male/female ratio, are evidence of an endocrine disruption effect. The guideline details the test protocol (method, duration, diet, etc.).

While this regulatory science is intended to assess risk and inform the normative decisions of regulatory agencies, the explanatory reports that accompany the guidelines highlight the innumerable difficulties and constraints of this assessment. These include the nonexistence of a "reliable model for overall environmental description", which leads to the provision of "rough estimates", even for the study of highly persistent compounds (OECD 2006a, p. 3); difficulties in extrapolating animal tests to humans; disagreements over the appropriate experimental model; the choice of exposure routes for testing a substance that does not correspond to actual human exposure to a combination of substances through more than one route (OECD 2006b, p. 2); and the impossibility of providing normative guidance (OECD 2013, p. 9).

Appendix II contains GLP, in other words, the standards that testing laboratories must apply for all nonclinical tests required by national regulations, for the registration or authorization of several products: pharmaceuticals, pesticides, food

16 A list of current and draft guidelines is available on the OECD website.

and feed additives, cosmetics, veterinary drugs and similar products, as well as for the regulation of industrial chemicals. The aim is to harmonize standards that apply to testing laboratories, so as to ensure the quality of test results. The OECD has subsequently supplemented these principles to ensure that test results are covered by a presumption of conformity to GLP principles.

Numerous other pesticide-specific tools complement the MAD. These include guidance documents, dossiers and reports on PPP authorization, residues, biopesticides, risk reduction, minor pesticide use, testing and assessment[17]. These documents are not legally binding, but this does not mean that they are not used by regulatory agencies and industry.

Regulatory science as described has been and continues to be developed by experts, not by the Council. They may be employed in both the public and industrial sectors. Among the references cited by the group of experts who prepared the MAD is a publication by the European Center for Ecotoxicology and Toxicology of Chemicals, a professional organization funded by the chemical industry. An OECD guideline document for conducting tests on occupational exposure to pesticides during their application (OECD 1997) was entirely written by an employee of Zeneca Agrochemicals[18] (Jouzel 2019, p. 157), which is worrying in terms of impartiality in the development of test methods. In reality, the entire body of regulatory science developed by the OECD since the 1970s needs to be investigated, in order to find out the extent of industrial participation in its development and the bias it may be affected by.

Today, the MAD is the equivalent of a multilateral agreement applicable in 45 countries[19]. Initially only applicable to OECD members, a decision taken in consideration of Chapter 19 of Agenda 21 (UNCED 1992) extended the MAD to nonmember countries in 1997. In view of the global goal of sustainable development set in Rio in 1992, the extension of the MAD has the aim of strengthening the ability of non-OECD countries that develop their own chemical industries to exchange information, ensuring that their chemical management systems do not lead to regulatory incompatibilities and the creation of trade barriers. With OECD members having to assess over 5,000 substances in large volumes, this expansion contributes to the objective of reducing the costs of chemical product management, as the

17 See: www.oecd.org/fr/securitechimique/pesticides-biocides/series-pesticides.htm [Accessed May 10, 2022].

18 In 1995, when Zeneca Agrochemicals employee G. Chester proposed the test method, the Anglo-Swedish company was producing chemicals including herbicides, fungicides and insecticides. In 2001, after Novartis and Monsanto, the company was the world's third-largest producer of agrochemicals.

19 In addition to OECD member countries bound by the MAD, other countries have joined the system: Argentina, Brazil, India, Malaysia, Singapore, South Africa and Thailand.

number of states sharing responsibility for testing increases. This is why the OECD has implemented a "proactive outreach strategy" (OECD 2010, p. 8).

The geographical coverage of the MAD, which contributes to its globalization, is also aided by the interplay of competition and cooperation between IOs. Since the 1970s, a number of IOs have taken up environmental issues, contributing to the fragmentation of international environmental law without, however, excluding circulation and permeability[20], particularly in the chemical sector. For example, the latest version of the International Code of Conduct on Pesticide Management refers to OECD GLP and some of its guidance documents (FAO and OMS 2014). In 1980, while the OECD presented itself as the "authority that was best placed" to harmonize chemical safety standards (OECD 1980, p. 13), three UN organizations created the first inter-agency cooperation program in the chemical sector, whose implementing agency, the World Health Organization (WHO), published documents for the assessment of chemical substances. This competitive situation was followed in 1995 by broader IO cooperation, with the OECD joining the Inter-Organization Program for the Sound Management of Chemicals. It was in this context that the Strategic Approach to International Chemicals Management (SAICM) was adopted in 2006, a nonbinding global policy initiative to minimize the adverse effects of chemicals. The SAICM, whose Global Action Plan contains measures to be achieved by 2020, calls for collaboration between the WHO and the OECD to develop and use new harmonized risk assessment methods, and to develop more effective methods and criteria for determining the impact of chemicals on human health. The nonbinding text refers to test guidelines, without mentioning OECD tools. Nevertheless, the OECD, which is responsible for more than 40% of the activities cited in the SAICM Global Action Plan (OECD 2010, p. 16), appears to be one of the main players in the measure in question. Ultimately, in the context of this international cooperation, the guidelines developed by the OECD are considered the most comprehensive set of international standards for the assessment of chemicals for regulatory purposes (UNEP 2019, p. 386). This inter-organizational cooperation is, of course, having an impact on the OECD, having adopted a binding decision for states to develop assessment methods together, without, however, obliging them to consider the risks arising from simultaneous exposure to several chemicals, which are the subject of a simple recommendation (OECD 2018).

4.3. The effects of the OECD's promotion of chemical safety ideas and tools in European law

The OECD's promotion of chemical safety ideas and tools has had at least two observable effects on European law. On the one hand, OECD regulatory science has

20 On these issues, see Maljean-Dubois (2017).

flowed into European law and, on the other, it has helped to generate ignorance[21] about the harmful effects of pesticides.

4.3.1. *The flow of regulatory science from the OECD to the European Union*

Under the terms of the first additional protocol to the OECD Convention, the European Communities established by the Treaties of Paris and Rome are represented at the OECD by the Commission. European texts concerning the MAD show that the EU adopts them in accordance with this OECD decision, without reference to any transposition into European law (Council of the European Union 1989; European Parliament and Council 2004). As a result of the EU's representation at the OECD and the legally binding nature of the first part of the MAD, the EU is bound by this text. However, the EU has clarified the nature of imported OECD texts: while the OECD guidelines are soft law for the EU, GLP is both soft and hard laws.

No general European act has been adopted to give legally binding power to the OECD guidelines as a whole. The first explicit reference in European law to the OECD guidelines appeared in 1984, in a text on the classification and labeling of hazardous substances (European Commission 1984). In 1994, a directive amending the one that was then applicable to the marketing of pesticides for agricultural use introduced three OECD guidelines into European law (European Commission 1994). It was not until 2009, in recital 58 of the PPP Regulation, that the EU affirmed the nonbinding nature of these guidelines. The text not only covers the OECD guidelines, but all "technical guidelines", since other institutions issue guidelines that are transposed into European law through an advisory procedure.

Two regulations implementing the PPP Regulation adopted in 2013 specify that "the list of test methods and guidance documents" are published in the Official Journal for "information" and "harmonization" purposes (European Commission 2013a, 2013b). There are two Commission communications that publish the specific lists of test methods to be implemented (European Commission 2013c, 2013d), including those of the OECD. In the typology of EU acts, these communications are nonlegislative acts implementing regulations. Consequently, the OECD guidelines did not acquire a legally binding nature when they were imported into European law. This means that the EU can disregard the OECD guidelines.

Over time, there have been numerous imports from the OECD, both in the general field of chemicals and in that of pesticides[22]. The communications issued for the implementation of the PPP Regulation mark a turning point in the introduction

21 At the heart of contemporary work in the social sciences, see Jouzel (2019).

22 The same applies to European regulations on cosmetics and animal feed additives.

of OECD standards into the European expert system, since they import them on a massive scale: 105 OECD guidelines have been Europeanized. In quantitative terms, OECD standards are the most numerous in European law[23], which supports the idea that OECD guidelines constitute the most comprehensive set of standards in the world. The Commission admits that this is due to a lack of expertise in Europe in the field of risk assessment regulation (European Commission 2001). There is no doubt that the European Economic Community, then the EU, shared the OECD's idea of developing world trade in chemical products in an economically efficient way, i.e. by limiting the cost of assessment. Perhaps, current European regulatory projects also reflect a genuine desire, on the one hand, to reduce the presence of chemical products, including pesticides, in our environment (European Commission 2020b), and, on the other, to develop the EU's capacity to develop and disseminate pesticide testing methods (European Commission 2022a).

GLP is now included in a European directive adopted in 2004 (European Parliament and Council 2004). The third article states that the Commission has the power to modify the principles of GLP, on "non-essential elements", in order to adapt them to technical progress. Measures adopted in this way constitute nonlegislative delegated acts within the meaning of Article 290 of the Treaty on the Functioning of the European Union. It follows that, under European law, GLP technical standards are not legally binding. On the other hand, other provisions relating to GLP are legally binding. For example, Article 1 of the Directive stipulates that member states must take measures to ensure that testing laboratories comply with the OECD principles of GLP appended to the Directive. Similarly, Article 3 of the Directive requires member states to adopt measures to monitor compliance with GLP principles, including "inspections and study checks in accordance with the recommendations of the OECD in this area".

4.3.2. *A regulatory science that produces ignorance*

The problem of assessing cumulative or cocktail effects is emblematic of the consequences of ideas and tools developed by the OECD but shared by the EU. The problem is not new. It was "an important shortcoming" of European law before the PPP Regulation was adopted (European Commission 2002, p. 15), and has been known about in the US since 1980 (Sprinkle and Payne-Sturges 2021).

---

23 Other guidelines for the assessment of PPPs in European law originate from the EU, including those issued by EFSA and the European Chemicals Agency, FAO, WHO, the European and Mediterranean Plant Protection Organization, the United Nations, the US Environmental Protection Agency and the Pest Management Regulatory Agency. Some test methods come from professional organizations, private entities such as ATSM, the European Seed Association, CropLife International and bodies whose members and laboratories are subsidiaries of world leaders in the agrochemical industry.

According to the PPP Regulation, chemical objects containing more than one substance are PPPs that are composed of "active substances, safeners or synergists" (Article 2.1), "preparations" defined as mixtures composed of two or more substances (Article 3.3), safeners, synergists, co-formulants and adjuvants, when they take the form of preparations (Article 2.3). Although the PPP Regulation expressly provides for synergists and safeners to be subject to the approval procedure, and stipulates that "data requirements [...] shall be defined" for these two categories of products (Article 25), the EU has still not adopted a regulation on testing methods specific to synergists and safeners that are not covered by the implementing regulations (European Commission 2013a, 2013b)[24] of the PPP Regulation, which were not updated until 2022 to take account of the inclusion of microorganisms in PPPs (European Commission 2022b, 2022c). This failure to act, which we emphasize has been going on for 13 years, may be explained by the fact that synergists and safeners can be mixtures or preparations for which the question of cumulative effects arises. The Commission acknowledges its inaction, which it justifies in two ways. In its view, as far as safeners are concerned, "serious adverse effects [...] seem unlikely", which sounds very much like a presumption of the absence of harmfulness that the CJEU unambiguously condemns (CJEU 2019, paragraph 80). The Commission goes on to explain that it has given priority to the inventory of unacceptable co-formulants, in view of resource constraints (European Commission 2020c, p. 3). In fact, it did not adopt the list of co-formulants that could not be used in PPPs until 2021, even though some member states had "identified" unacceptable co-formulants in PPPs authorized under the pre-PPP rules, in other words, between 1991 and 2009 (European Commission 2021, p. 8). The Commission also notes that the authorization procedures for adjuvants, for which Article 58 of the PPP Regulation lays down data requirements, have still not been adopted (European Commission 2021, p. 8). Contrary to the letter of the PPP Regulation, synergists, safeners and adjuvants are therefore included in the composition of PPPs placed on the market without any prior European assessment of each of these three chemical categories, whether they come in the form of a single substance or a mixture of substances, and this was also the case for co-formulants until 2021.

With regard to PPPs, the PPP Regulation stipulates that an active substance is approved at the European level "in the light of current scientific and technical knowledge", if it is foreseeable that the PPP containing this substance has no harmful effect on human or animal health, "taking into account known cumulative and synergistic effects" (Article 4). Other provisions reinforce the obligation to assess cocktail effects, such as Article 29.6 of the PPP Regulation, which states that the "interaction between the active substance, safeners, synergists and co-formulants shall be taken into account during the evaluation". A regulation implementing the PPP Regulation specifies that the information to be produced by manufacturers so as

24 They only concern active substances and PPPs.

to enable the PPP to be assessed must include information on the "potentially harmful effects" of the PPP on human and animal health, groundwater, the "potentially unacceptable effects [...] on the environment, on plants and plant products", "as well as known and expected cumulative and synergistic effects" (European Commission 2013b, Appendix, paragraphs 1.1–1.3). Lastly, Article 4 of the PPP Regulation states that the active substance is approved at the European level if, "having regard to realistic conditions of use", the residues of the PPP containing it and the PPP itself have no harmful effect on health or the environment. This means that the cocktail effect on the environment, in other words, where the PPP is actually used, must first be assessed when the active substance is approved by the European authorities. Nevertheless, Article 4 of the PPP Regulation contains a precautionary wording in its requirement to assess cumulative effects, since it specifies that they are taken into account "where the scientific methods accepted by" EFSA "to assess such effects are available". This is precisely the flaw in European law, since EFSA has still not agreed on a method for this purpose, even though the problem has been known since at least 2002, i.e. 20 years of exposure of human and animal populations to chemical cocktails. Once again, the Commission justifies this inaction, this time on the grounds of greater complexity than initially envisaged, and announces the development of an assessment method, an action plan to set priorities for ongoing work, and calls for research projects on methods for assessing cumulative risks to ecosystems (Commission 2020c, p. 9 and p. 11). It is true that the European Parliament, NGOs and scientists are denouncing this situation and sometimes proposing solutions, but for the time being and despite a longstanding knowledge of the issue, European regulatory science is conspicuous by its ignorance of these effects. Although the CJEU, questioned by Tribunal correctionnel de Foix (the Foix criminal court), ruled that the assessment of an active substance "cannot be carried out in an objective fashion while failing to take into account the effects deriving from a possible combination of various constituents" of a PPP, adding that this requirement applies to both EFSA and the Member States, it disregarded EFSA's failure to accept the assessment method, concluding that the PPP Regulation was not tainted by an evident error of assessment (CJEU 2019, paragraphs 62–76). Perhaps, the Court should be asked about the lack of a regulatory method for assessing cumulative effects, and the possibility of taking account, at least on a transitional basis, of such methods proposed in academic publications, particularly in light of Article 4.1 of the PPP Regulation, which does not require the assessment to be carried out on the basis of a regulatory science, but solely with regard to the "current state of scientific and technical knowledge", in order to ensure that the cumulative effect in a complex product and in the environment does not meet any of the exclusion criteria for the approval of a substance, in other words, an effect that it is neither mutagenic, carcinogenic, toxic for reproduction, nor endocrine disruptive. However, the observation of cocktail effects in the environment presupposes that the latter is carefully monitored. However, as the European Court of Auditors points out, this monitoring, which is a complementary warning system to the assessment, has many shortcomings, partly due to the inadequacy of texts on statistics and the sustainable use of pesticides (Council of the European Union 2020, pp. 28–35).

As for the OECD, it is working to develop methods for testing cocktail effects, drawing on those developed by the US Environmental Protection Agency (EPA) between 1999 and 2006 (OECD 2017). Unsurprisingly, the EPA's 2003 definition of cumulative effects has been circulated to EFSA (2020a, p. 7; 2020b, p. 6), whose relevance is contested for various reasons: because it is based on the assessment of dose additivity, with a common mechanism of toxicity rather than on the interaction, synergism and antagonism between substances, without considering the community vulnerability, the multiplicity of exposure routes and other available methods, including epidemiological models (Sprinkle and Payne-Sturges 2021). Moreover, such a definition goes against the PPP Regulation, which expressly determines the assessment of "cumulative and synergistic effects" (Article 4).

4.4. Conclusion

As European law currently stands, the obligation to assess cocktail effects exists, but the EU's inaction on synergists, safeners, adjuvants and PPPs renders it ineffective, confirming scientists' observation that the production of chemical products is outstripping the world's capacity for assessment and monitoring. Numerous other examples that cannot be discussed here illustrate the gray areas created by the European expert system. The European Parliament has noted this and emphasized the need to take account of non-regulatory scientific literature, which should have the same "probative value" in assessment as studies based on GLP (European Parliament and Council 2019). In addition to this, the European Ombudsman, who was twice called upon to assess certain substance approval practices by the Commission, supports this observation (European Ombudsman 2016, 2020).

As an epilogue, the OECD wrote the following half a century ago:

> The presence of a chemical in the environment may adversely affect man by chronically exposing him to the chemical or by causing the deterioration of materials and biological systems which are beneficial to his survival. Contamination of the environment by cumulative pollutants is of particular concern due to the insidious nature of the process and the difficulty of correcting any damage that may have occurred (OECD 1974, explanatory note, point 4).

In spite of this, the choice has been made to commit to a deadly path by placing the law at the service of chemical market development, and the current observation of regulatory inability to prevent the destruction of the common home does not prevent chemical production from growing until 2060 (OECD 2019, p. 6; UNEP 2019, p. 27).

MAD: Mutual Acceptance of Data in the Assessment of Chemicals

GLP: Good Laboratory Practice

CJEU: Court of Justice of the European Union

OECD: Organisation for Economic Cooperation and Development

IO: international organization

OPECST: Office parlementaire d'évaluation des choix scientifiques et technologiques (French Parliamentary Office for the Evaluation of Scientific and Technological Choices)

SFDI: Société française pour le droit international (French Society for International Law)

EGC: European General Court

Box 4.1. *Summary of acronyms*

4.5. References

Bonvallot, N., Brimo, S., Boudes, P., Coumoul, X., Duboc, S., Mougin, C., Salles, B. (2021). Pour une gestion alerte du risque chimique – risques (éco)toxicologiques pour les êtres humains et l'environnement dans une logique de biodiversité. Report, cnDAspe, Paris.

Carson, R. (1962). *Silent Spring*. Houghton Mifflin Company, Boston.

CJEU (2019). Arrêt de la Cour (grande chambre) du 1er octobre 2019. Document, 62017CJ0616.

Council of the European Union (1978a). Directive 78/631/CEE du 26 juin concernant le rapprochement des législations des États membres relatives à la classification, l'emballage et l'étiquetage des préparations dangereuses (pesticides). *Journal officiel des Communautés européennes*, L 206, 13–25.

Council of the European Union (1978b). Directive 79/117/CEE du 21 décembre, concernant l'interdiction de mise sur le marché et d'utilisation des produits phytopharmaceutiques contenant certaines substances actives. *Journal officiel des Communautés européennes*, L 33/36, 36–40.

Council of the European Union (1989). Décision du 28 juillet concernant l'acceptation par la Communauté économique européenne d'une décision-recommandation de l'OCDE sur la mise en conformité aux principes de bonnes pratiques de laboratoire. *Official Journal of the European Union*, L 315/1, 1–32.

Council of the European Union (1991). Directive 91/414/CEE du 15 juillet concernant la mise sur le marché des produits phytopharmaceutiques. *Journal officiel des Communautés européennes*, L 230, 1–32.

Council of the European Union (2020). Utilisation durable des produits phytopharmaceutiques : des progrès limités en matière de mesure et de réduction des risques. Report, Council of the European Union, Brussels.

Council of the European Union (2021). Décision (UE) 2021/764 du 10 mai établissant le programme spécifique d'exécution du programme-cadre pour la recherche et l'innovation "Horizon Europe", et abrogeant la décision 2013/743/UE. *Official Journal of the European Union*, LI 167/1, 1–80.

Demortain, D. (2017). Expertise, regulatory science and the evaluation of technology and risk: Introduction to the special issue. *Minerva*, 55(2), 139–159.

Demortain, D. and Borraz, O. (2015). Science réglementaire. In *Dictionnaire critique de l'expertise. Santé, travail, environnement*, Gilbert, C., Henry, E., Jouzel, J.-N., Marichalar, P. (eds). Presses de Sciences Po, Paris.

EFSA (2020a). Cumulative dietary risk characterisation of pesticides that have acute effects on the nervous system. *EFSA Journal*, 18(4), 6087.

EFSA (2020b). Cumulative dietary risk characterisation of pesticides that have chronic effects on the thyroid. *EFSA Journal*, 18(4), 6088.

EGC (2015). Judgment of 16th December. Suède/Commission, Document 61960CJ0006.

EGC (2016). Judgment of 20th September. PAN Europe/Commission, Document 61999CJ0184.

European Commission (1984). Commission Directive 84/449/EEC of 25 April 1984 adapting to technical progress for the sixth time Council Directive 67/548/EEC on the approximation of laws, regulations and administrative provisions relating to the classification, packaging and labelling of dangerous substances. *Official Journal of the European Union*, L 251, 1–223 [Online]. Available at: https://op.europa.eu/publication-detail/-/publication/66fbfb15-9c2c-49d3-bf1b-39075bdb56dc.

European Commission (1994). Directive 94/37/CE du 22 juillet modifiant la directive 91/414/CEE du Conseil concernant la mise sur le marché des produits phytopharmaceutiques, 29 July. *Official Journal of the European Union*, L 194, 65–81.

European Commission (2001). Evaluation of the active substances of plant protection products (submitted in accordance with Article 8(2) of Council Directive 91/414/EEC on the placing of plant protection products on the market). Report, European Commission, Brussels.

European Commission (2002). Towards a thematic strategy on the sustainable use of pesticides, COM(2002)349 final. Report, European Commission, Brussels.

European Commission (2013a). Commission Regulation (EU) No 283/2013 of 1 March 2013 setting out the data requirements for active substances, in accordance with Regulation (EC) No 1107/2009 of the European Parliament and of the Council concerning the placing of plant protection products on the market. *Official Journal of the European Union*, L 93, 1–84.

European Commission (2013b). Commission Regulation (EU) No 284/2013 of 1 March 2013 setting out the data requirements for plant protection products, in accordance with Regulation (EC) No 1107/2009 of the European Parliament and of the Council concerning the placing of plant protection products on the market. *Official Journal of the European Union*, L 93, 85–152.

European Commission (2013c). Commission Communication in the framework of the implementation of Commission Regulation (EU) No 283/2013 of 1 March 2013 setting out the data requirements for active substances, in accordance with Regulation (EC) No 1107/2009 of the European Parliament and of the Council concerning the placing of plant protection products on the market. *Official Journal of the European Union*, C 95/1, 1–20.

European Commission (2013d). Communication from the Commission in the framework of the implementation of Part A of the Annex of the Commission Regulation (EU) No 284/2013 setting out the data requirements for plant protection products, in accordance with Regulation (EC) No 1107/2009 of the European Parliament and of the Council concerning the placing of plant protection products on the market. *Official Journal of the European Union*, C 344, 1–36.

European Commission (2020a). Pharmaceutical Strategy for Europe, COM(2020)761 final. Report, European Commission, Brussels

European Commission (2020b). Chemicals Strategy for Sustainability. Towards a Toxic-Free Environment, COM(2020)667 final. Report, European Commission, Brussels.

European Commission (2020c). Evaluation of Regulation (EC) No 1107/2009 on the placing of plant protection products on the market and of Regulation (EC) No 396/2005 on maximum residue levels of pesticides, COM(2020)208 final. Report, European Commission, Brussels [Online]. Available at: https://eur-lex.europa.eu/legal-content/EN/TXT/PDF/?uri=CELEX:52020DC0208&qid=1716369936624.

European Commission (2021). Commission Regulation (EU) 2021/383 of 3 March 2021 amending Annex III to Regulation (EC) No 1107/2009 of the European Parliament and of the Council listing co-formulants which are not accepted for inclusion in plant protection products. *Official Journal of the European Union*, L 74, 7–26.

European Commission (2022a). An EU Strategy on Standardisation Setting global standards in support of a resilient, green and digital EU single market, COM(2022)31 final. Report, European Commission, Brussels.

European Commission (2022b). Commission Regulation (EU) 2022/1439 of 31 August 2022 amending Regulation (EU) No 283/2013 as regards the information to be submitted for active substances and the specific data requirements for micro-organisms. *Official Journal of the European Union*, L 227, 8–37.

European Commission (2022c). Commission Regulation (EU) 2022/1440 of 31 August 2022 amending Regulation (EU) No 284/2013 as regards the information to be submitted for plant protection products and the specific data requirements for plant protection products containing micro-organisms. *Official Journal of the European Union*, L 227, 38–69.

European Ombudsman (2016). Decision in case 12/2013/MDC on the practices of the European Commission regarding the authorisation and placing on the market of plant protection products (pesticides). Case 12/2013/MDC, European Ombudsman, Belgium.

European Ombudsman (2020). Decision in joint cases 1570/2018/JF-JN and 1973/2018/JF-JN on how the European Commission approves substances used in plant protection products (pesticides). Case 1570/2018/JF, European Ombudsman, Belgium.

European Ombudsman (2021). Decision on how the European Commission involved stakeholders and managed conflicts of interest in reviewing the protection goals for assessing environmental risks of pesticides. Case 1402/2020/TE, European Ombudsman, Belgium.

European Parliament and Council (2004). Directive 2004/10/EC of the European Parliament and of the Council of 11 February 2004 on the harmonisation of laws, regulations and administrative provisions relating to the application of the principles of good laboratory practice and the verification of their applications for tests on chemical substances (codified version). *Official Journal of the European Union*, L 50/44, 44–59 [Online]. Available at: https://eur-lex.europa.eu/legal-content/EN/TXT/?uri=CELEX%3A02004L0010-20090420&qid=1725976620258.

European Parliament and Council (2006). Regulation (EC) No 1907/2006 of the European Parliament and of the Council of 18 December 2006 concerning the Registration, Evaluation, Authorisation and Restriction of Chemicals (REACH), establishing a European Chemicals Agency, amending Directive 1999/45/EC and repealing Council Regulation (EEC) No 793/93 and Commission Regulation (EC) No 1488/94 as well as Council Directive 76/769/EEC and Commission Directives 91/155/EEC, 93/67/EEC, 93/105/EC and 2000/21/EC. *Official Journal of the European Union*, L 396, 1–849.

European Parliament and Council (2009a). Regulation (EC) No 1107/2009 of the European Parliament and of the Council of 21 October 2009 concerning the placing of plant protection products on the market and repealing Council Directives 79/117/EEC and 91/414/EEC. *Official Journal of the European Union*, L 309, 1–50.

European Parliament and Council (2009b). Directive 2009/128/EC of the European Parliament and of the Council of 21 October 2009 establishing a framework for Community action to achieve the sustainable use of pesticides. *Official Journal of the European Union*, L 309/71, 71–86.

European Parliament and Council (2019). European Parliament resolution of 16 January 2019 on the Union's authorisation procedure for pesticides (2018/2153(INI)). *Official Journal of the European Union*, C 411/48, 48–67.

FAO and OMS (2014). The International Code of Conduct on Pesticide Management. Report, Food and Agriculture Organization of the United Nations and World Health Orgnization, Rome.

Gérard, M. (2020). La FAO se rapproche du lobby des pesticides, 22 November. *Le Monde* [Online]. Available at: https://www.lemonde.fr/planete/article/2020/11/20/le-rapprochement-entre-la-fao-et-le-lobby-des-pesticides-inquiete-scientifiques-et-ong_6060582_3244.html.

Horel, S. (2015). *Intoxication. Perturbateurs endocriniens, lobbyistes et eurocrates : une bataille d'influence contre la santé*. La Découverte, Paris.

Jones, M.M. and Benrubi, I.D. (2013). Poison politics: A contentious history of consumer protection against dangerous household chemicals in the United States. *American Journal of Public Health*, 103(5), 801–812.

Jouzel, J.N. (2019). *Pesticides. Comment ignorer ce que l'on sait*. Presses de Sciences Po, Paris.

Maljean-Dubois, S. (ed.) (2017). *Circulations de normes et réseaux d'acteurs dans la gouvernance internationale de l'environnement*. Confluence des droits, Aix-en-Provence.

Meyer, J.H. (2017). Who should pay for pollution? The OECD, the European Communities and the emergence of environmental policy in the early 1970s. *European Review of History*, 24(3), 377–398.

OECD (1960). Convention on the organisation for economic co-operation and development [Online]. Available at: https://www.oecd.org/en/about/legal/text-of-the-convention-on-the-organisation-for-economic-co-operation-and-development.html.

OECD (1972). Recommendation of the council on guiding principles concerning international economic aspects of environmental policies. OECD/LEGAL/0102 [Online]. Available at: https://legalinstruments.oecd.org/en/instruments/OECD-LEGAL-0102.

OECD (1974). Recommendation of the council on the assessment of the potential environmental effects of chemicals. OECD/LEGAL/0135 [Online]. Available at: https://legalinstruments.oecd.org/en/instruments/OECD-LEGAL-0135.

OECD (1977a). Recommendation of the council establishing guidelines in respect of procedure and requirements for anticipating the effects of chemicals on man and in the environment. OECD/LEGAL/0154 [Online]. Available at: https://legalinstruments.oecd.org/en/instruments/OECD-LEGAL-0154.

OECD (1977b). *L'évaluation des effets potentiels des produits chimiques dans l'environnement*. OECD, Paris.

OECD (1980). *Réunion à haut niveau du groupe des produits chimiques*. OECD, Paris.

OECD (1981). Decision of the council concerning the mutual acceptance of data in the assessment of chemicals. Legal Instruments, OECD/LEGAL/0194, Paris [Online]. Available at: https://legalinstruments.oecd.org/en/instruments/OECD-LEGAL-0194.

OECD (1987). Decision-recommendation of the council on the systematic investigation of existing chemicals. Legal Instruments, OECD/LEGAL/0232, Paris [Online]. Available at: https://legalinstruments.oecd.org/en/instruments/OECD-LEGAL-0232.

OECD (1997). *Guidance Document for the Conduct of Studies of Occupational Exposure to Pesticides during Agricultural Application*. OECD, Paris.

OECD (2006a). Summary of Considerations in the Report from the OECD Expert Group on Physical Chemistry. OECD, Paris [Online]. Available at: https://www.oecd-ilibrary.org/environment/summary-of-considerations-in-the-report-from-the-oecd-expert-group-on-physical-chemistry_9789264013391-en.

OECD (2006b). Summary of Considerations in the Report from the OECD Expert Groups on Short Term and Long Term Toxicology. OECD, Paris [Online]. Available at: https://www.oecd-ilibrary.org/environment/summary-of-considerations-in-the-report-from-the-oecd-expert-groups-on-short-term-and-long-term-toxicology_9789264035447-en.

OECD (2010). Cutting Costs in Chemicals Management. OECD, Paris [Online]. Available at: https://www.oecd-ilibrary.org/environment/cutting-costs-in-chemicals-management_9789264085930-en.

OECD (2011a). *Le comité des politiques d'environnement célèbre ses 40 ans d'activités. 1971–2011*. OECD, Paris.

OECD (2011b). *40 Years of Chemical Safety at the OECD: Quality and Efficiency*. OECD, Paris.

OECD (2012). OECD Environmental Outlook to 2050: The Consequences of Inaction. OECD, Paris [Online]. Available at: https://www.oecd-ilibrary.org/environment/oecd-environmental-outlook-to-2050_9789264122246-en.

OECD (2013). OECD Guidelines for the Testing of Chemicals, Section 5. OECD, Paris.

OECD (2015). *Preliminary Analysis of Policy Drivers Influencing Decision Making in Chemicals Management*. OECD, Paris.

OECD (2017). *Case Study on the Use of Integrated Approaches for Testing and Assessment for Pesticide Cumulative Risk Assessment & Assessment of Lifestage Susceptibility*. OECD, Paris.

OECD (2018). Decision-Recommendation of the Council on the Co-operative Investigation and Risk Reduction of Chemicals. Legal instruments, OECD/LEGAL/0441, Paris [Online]. Available at: https://legalinstruments.oecd.org/en/instruments/OECD-LEGAL-0441.

OECD (2019). *OECD Work on Chemical Safety and Biosafety*. OECD, Paris.

OPECST (2021). Le déclin des insectes. *Les notes scientifiques de l'office*, 30 [Online]. Available at: http://www.senat.fr/rap/r21-286/r21-2861.pdf [Accessed 12 January 2022].

Persson, L., Carney Almroth, B.M., Collins, C.D., Cornell, S., de Wit, C.A., Diamond, M.L., Fantke, P., Hassellöv, M., MacLeod, M., Ryberg, M.W. et al. (2022). Outside the safe operating space of the planetary boundary for novel entities. *Environmental Science & Technology*, 56(3), 1510–1521.

Rockström, J., Steffen, W., Noone, K., Persson, A., Stuart, F., Lambin, E., Lenton, M.T., Scheffer, M., Folke, C., Schellnhuber, H.J. et al. (2009). Planetary boundaries: Exploring the safe operating space for humanity. *Ecology and Society*, 14(2), 32.

SFDI (2013). *Le pouvoir normatif de l'OCDE*. Pédone, Paris.

Sprinkle, R.H. and Payne-Sturges, D.C. (2021). Mixture toxicity, cumulative risk, and environmental justice in United States federal policy, 1980–2016. *Environmental Health*, 20(104). doi: 10.1186/s12940-021-00764-5.

UNCED (1992). Chapter 19 of Agenda 21 programme. In *United Nations Conference on Environment & Development*, 3–14 June. United Nations, Rio de Janerio, [Online]. Available at: https://sustainabledevelopment.un.org/content/documents/Agenda21.pdf?_gl=1*382enn*_ga*MTMwNTQyNDYzMS4xNzI1NTI3Nzk2*_ga_TK9BQL5X7Z*MTcyNTk2OTI3My4yLjEuMTcyNTk2OTQ3MC4wLjAuMA [Accessed 10 September 2024].

UNEP (2019). Global chemicals outlook II – From legacies to innovative solutions: Implementing the 2030 agenda for sustainable development. United Nations Environment Programme, Nairobi.

5

Fighting the Colorado Potato Beetle in Francoist Spain (1939–1953)

5.1. Introduction

At the start of the 21st century, Spain became one of Europe's biggest consumers of pesticides, whereas their use in Spanish agriculture was marginal during the first half of the 20th century. During the interwar years, agricultural engineers angrily lamented the occasional use of fertilizers and pesticides, calling for more to be used. Statistical data analyzed by González de Molina et al. (2020) show that there was a sharp increase during the 1970s and 1980s, but there are still uncertainties about earlier decades. Indeed, it is difficult to calculate these variations quantitatively, not only because of the disparity of available data but also because of the diversity of plant protection products, fluctuating prices and the quantities required for each pesticide, which introduces difficulties for long-term comparisons (González de Molina et al. 2020, pp. 96–98).

To overcome the methodological obstacles presented by the scarcity of quantified data, we adopt a qualitative perspective, drawing on a variety of historical sources, in order to explore the issues surrounding pesticide use in Franco's Spain. The aim is twofold: firstly, to shed light on the use of large quantities of hazardous pesticides during the early years of Franco's dictatorship and secondly, to propose elements of explanation for this phenomenon, linked to the convergence of a series of ecological, political and economic factors. Ecological factors include the arrival of a new insect (the Colorado potato beetle, which we shall return to in section 5.4), which affected the production of potatoes, one of the main agricultural products during these years. In this analysis, we also take into account the agricultural modernization projects and autarky policies that characterized the early years of

---

Chapter written by José Ramón BERTOMEU SÁNCHEZ.

Franco's government, as well as attempts to create a national pesticide industry. With regard to the latter, the period was marked by a shift from arsenic-based products to organochlorines (including DDT), which provided alternative ways of combating "harmful" insects in a new political and economic context since World War II.

This case study will enable us to reflect on the historical ontology of pesticides, which stems from their dual political and material nature (Bertomeu Sánchez 2019a; Boudia et al. 2021). These are products whose emergence was enabled by social and cultural practices during the early years of Franco's dictatorship. Particular attention is paid to the visible and invisible violence associated with pesticides, as well as to the more or less explicit forms of coercion which produced a risk/benefit ratio that was favorable to the most powerful groups of the new regime. The history of pesticides thus provides keys to understanding important aspects of the early Francoist dictatorship, while analysis of this context raises questions about how to think about this crucial decade, marked by the advent of pesticides in the fields of agriculture, public health and domestic use (Pérez Criado and Bertomeu Sánchez 2020). This study offers new insights into the use of pesticides through the prism of ignorance studies, environmental justice and toxic violence.

From a historical perspective, this chapter covers the first two decades of Franco's dictatorship (1936–1977), the regime established after the military coup against the Second Spanish Republic in 1936, which launched the Spanish Civil War. The early 1940s were marked by autarky policies, the strong influence of fascist groups such as Falange, and brutal repression against dissidents, especially defenders of the old Republic. The situation persisted until at least 1944, when the end of World War II and the fall of fascist governments in Europe brought the Franco regime to a certain degree of international isolation. With inaccurate and contested temporary limits, it is customary to consider this "first Franco regime" as lasting until the mid-1950s, with a new generation of Franco politicians in power and a more dynamic economy in an international context, marked by both the Cold War and cooperation with the United States.

The main sources analyzed in this chapter are the archives of the Ministry of Agriculture, available in the General Administration Archive. These include reports and accounts written by agricultural engineers on the control of major pests, published annually for all Spanish provinces. We have also explored local archives which record both specific agricultural activities in the fields, as well as the reaction of anonymous farmers and political authorities. Studies published in academic agricultural engineering journals and in the agricultural and general press, in which numerous details of Colorado potato beetle control activities are recorded, were also used.

This chapter is divided into five parts. Section 5.2 provides an overview of international studies on the subject of pesticides, followed by section 5.3 on the autarky policies of the early Franco governments, which encouraged the use of arsenic pesticides as the sole means of controlling the Colorado potato beetle. Section 5.4 focuses on this struggle and the crucial role played by agricultural engineers in articulating agrarian modernization projects with the policies of the new authoritarian regime. Using the province of Burgos as an example, we analyze the communication campaigns aimed at overcoming farmers' resistance. Section 5.5 deals with the arrival of DDT against a backdrop of numerous decrees issued by the Franco government to regulate the production and use of pesticides. Section 5.6 analyzes how this legal architecture encouraged the production and consumption of pesticides, while the toxic risks to the population and the environment were largely neglected.

5.2. The technopolitics of pesticides

For several years now, a field of study has been emerging around the history of toxic products such as asbestos, lead, mercury, arsenic, pesticides, endocrine disruptors and many other chemicals. These products have been analyzed in a variety of spaces, including workplaces and homes, industries, farms and agricultural operations, air and rivers, etc. These analyses consider historical actors, forms of regulation and heterogeneous scales of analysis. Many of these studies are inspired by the desire to cross disciplinary barriers and enter the public debate with new narratives and perspectives for thinking about a world which has become toxic[1].

It is then necessary to think of these toxic products as sociomaterial entities beyond the dichotomies of nature and culture, science and politics (Boudia et al. 2021). In early Francoist Spain, pesticides were introduced by agricultural engineers who took advantage of the political rhetoric on autarky. At the same time, policies to eradicate the Colorado potato beetle helped establish the dictatorship's control over the rural world; it was therefore a question of co-production between industry, agriculture and the authoritarian social order (Jasanoff 2004; Saraiva 2016).

In addition to the links between the political regime and pest control, a perspective focused on the practices of creation of ignorance (the range of issues associated with the new discipline of "agnotology") seems to be relevant to this research. Toxic products circulate in networks for the production of knowledge and ignorance, which make toxic risks visible or invisible, thereby encouraging different types of collective action or public inaction. The circulation of ignorance is likely to delay risk control, weaken regulations and shift the burden of toxic damages onto certain groups: rural

1 A summary of the academic literature is provided in Bertomeu Sánchez (2020b).

communities, farm workers and food consumers (Proctor and Schiebinger 2008; Kourany and Carrier 2020). Studies of "undone science" highlight structural issues such as institutional frameworks that discourage the production and circulation of data considered to be "sensitive" by political and economic powers (Boudia and Henry 2022). Even when there is sufficient data on the hazardous nature of products, the circulation of this toxicological knowledge is limited to academic circles, without reaching the decision-making or public debate spaces. In this way, it is possible to "ignore what we know" in pesticide regulations (Jouzel 2019) or to "underestimate" the risks associated with pesticides, due to a lack of epidemiological data (Dedieu et al. 2015).

Paradoxically, the vast literature on the history of pesticides has contributed to the invisibility of certain aspects of the problem. The first studies focused on DDT in the United States, the disappearance of the American eagle, the debates surrounding Rachel Carson's *Silent Spring* (1962) and the rise of the citizens' movement that led to the banning of DDT. This apparent success contributed to the neglect of other products (arsenic or organophosphate pesticides), the invisibility of other dangers (occupational hazards, food safety) and other categories of victims (rural communities, farm workers). To avoid these "synecdoche problems", historian Frederic R. Davis called for the development of a "synthetic approach", integrating elements of the history of science and environmental history (Davis 2019).

Among the new works helping to account for the complexity of the problem, we can mention those on the use of pesticides by the British Empire (Clarke 2012), on the close relationship between these industries and the British government (Clarke and Lean 2022), as well as those focusing on advertising campaigns to facilitate the use of DDT in the United States (Mart 2015; Conis 2022). The precarious situation of workers, particularly women, and their ways of acting against toxic risks are new angles in this blooming research (Guthman 2019).

In Latin America, the fight against glyphosate fumigation has fostered various forms of resistance in countries such as Colombia (Lyons 2018, 2020) and Argentina (Arancibia and Motta 2019). In Mexico, the circulation of temporary agricultural workers and the pressure of the international food market have created conditions of invisible intoxication (Wright 2005), while the role of government institutions has fueled confusion between producers and regulators (Bravo et al. 2020).

On the European continent, numerous studies have been devoted to the health problems of agricultural workers and rural communities, notably in France (Jas 2007; Dedieu et al. 2015; Jouzel 2019). In Spain, the history of pesticides was initially written through the prism of progress narratives, supported by the main actors who contributed to their diffusion (Cano Manuel 1979). In addition, some science historians have highlighted and even celebrated the contributions of Spanish chemists to the synthesis of organochlorine pesticides (Andrés Turrión 2019). Historical research on 20th-century Spain has only recently begun to take the agnotological perspective into account, focusing on hydrocyanic acid fumigation in the first half of the century (Guillem Llobat 2019), the use of arsenic pesticides during the early Franco regime (Bertomeu Sánchez 2019) and the emergence of new practices and sociotechnical imaginaries after the arrival of DDT (Pérez Criado and Bertomeu Sánchez 2020). Moreover, new research has been conducted on the production and use of other organochlorine pesticides such as lindane, which caused serious public health and environmental problems (Pérez 2022). Other recent publications have provided fresh perspectives on the translation and reception of Rachel Carson's book *Silent Spring* (Pérez Criado 2017). This chapter follows in the wake of this research, while integrating recent reflections around science, technology and agriculture in Francoist Spain[2].

5.3. Autarky and arsenic pesticides

Although little studied, the history of pesticides prior to World War II goes back a long way. The period preceding the advent of DDT was characterized by the use of mineral compounds and natural product extracts. In the mid-19th century, new products were introduced, such as copper-based fungicides (the best-known is the Bordeaux mixture, a copper sulfate solution) and arsenic compounds (Paris green and lead arsenate, which will be discussed later). These were later partially replaced by synthetic organic compounds such as DDT and other organochlorines such as lindane and organophosphates, which appeared after World War II. In the 1960s, agronomists had a wide variety of products at their disposal.

Introduced in the late 19th century in the United States, lead arsenate was one of the arsenic products used to control pests in the first third of the 20th century (Whorton 1974; Spear 2005). It was used alongside other arsenic insecticides such as Paris green or calcium arsenate to combat the growing number of pests caused by the rise of monocultures and transnational food trade. Arsenic was a by-product of the metallurgical chemical industry, which could be used in agriculture, becoming a profitable way of disposing of toxic industrial waste (Romero 2021).

Other procedures were explored in the first half of the 20th century, such as biological control, research into pest-resistant crops and modifications to cultivation techniques. However, the growing availability of industrial wastes (such as arsenics)

2 Many issues have been revisited in recent years: agricultural technologies (Fernández Prieto 2014), hydraulic engineering (Swyngedouw 2015), "Franco's engineers" (Camprubí Bueno 2017) and Spanish chemistry (Nieto-Galan 2019).

and the development of the organic pesticide industry in the second half of the century have made chemical control the main – and sometimes the only – method of combating agricultural pests and diseases transmitted by insects or fungi. The use of arsenic pesticides has led to debates about health and food risks, particularly following cases of collective intoxication and commercial controversies[3].

Lead arsenate arrived in Spain at the beginning of the 20th century, as in other countries such as France and Germany[4]. It was used to combat various problems affecting vines, olives and apples. Consumption was very low before the 1940s, as it was an expensive imported product, given the weakness of the Spanish chemical industry. In 1934, the General Directorate of Agriculture requested that the import of pesticides be facilitated, with a view to reducing costs. The list of products requested illustrates the types of pesticides that were most commonly used in Spain at the time: a few plant-originated products (nicotine, pyrethrum, derris, various oils), most being mineral substances such as copper compounds (the chemical base for making Bordeaux mixture and other pesticides), cyanides (for fumigations) or arsenic compounds, including lead arsenate[5].

The outbreak of World War II brought pesticide imports to a halt. Geologists, agronomists and other experts thought that it was necessary to wait for the end of the war and the return of imports to continue production of this group of mineral pesticides, but the reopening of arsenic mines in the north of the Iberian Peninsula changed the situation. Thus, with the help of the geologists, Franco's various governments encouraged domestic production of arsenic pesticides as a paradigmatic example of autarky policies. They also encouraged the creation of national industries with a mandatory pesticide register, thus imposing quality control against fraud. This reduced the number of authorizations for distributors of foreign products, which were subject to stricter standards.

5.4. Controlling the Colorado beetle

Before discussing regulations, it is necessary to describe other non-human factors that encouraged the use of pesticides during the early years of Francoist dictatorship: the Colorado potato beetle (*Leptinotarsa decemlineata*). Native to the central United States, it arrived on the West Coast at the end of the 19th century and, with the help

3 For debates surrounding the use of arsenic insecticides in France, see Fourche (2017). There are two examples of poisoning in Phillips and French (1998) and Suay Matallana and Guillem Llobat (2018).

4 See the works by Fourche (2004), Spear (2005), Straumann (2005, pp. 164–170) and Saraiva (2016, pp. 87–90).

5 Administration Archives (AGA), 61/768. Pest Section, Madrid. September 18, 1934.

of transatlantic ships, reached Europe in the 1920s[6]. The rise of railroads and the expansion of potato monocultures also contributed to its dispersion. European governments implemented drastic measures to contain the pest: crop burning, protection zones, surveillance systems and massive fumigation of affected areas. Despite this, the beetle continued to spread from western France to the Pyrenees, where the first outbreaks were discovered in the mid-1930s (Cañizo 1928, 1932; Alfaro Moreno 1945).

The risk to potato production has been highlighted by entomologists in several countries, including Spain. In fact, as early as 1877, naturalist and forestry engineer Esteban Boutelou Soldevilla (1877) noted that the potato beetle could cause a food crisis equal to or worse than the great famine caused in north-western Europe by late blight in previous decades. He recommended a series of actions to combat the insect: the "multiplication of its natural enemies and parasites", the manual collection of larvae and adults and, finally, arsenic insecticides, notably Paris green, which were commonly used before the arrival of lead arsenate. In addition to identifying the threat, Boutelou's work shows that a whole range of pest control methods were available, pesticides being just one of them.

The first case in the Iberian Peninsula was detected in Massanet de Cabrenys (Girona) in the summer of 1935. The measures adopted seemed to contain the plague, but the disorder caused by Franco's military coup and the ensuing war prevented containment actions, aimed at containing its spread. With the disorganization of agronomic services caused by the civil war, there was a lack of control of the plague and new outbreaks appeared (Alfaro Moreno 1945). One of the agronomists who coordinated the pest control services described the challenges of the first years of the 1940s as follows: shortage of pesticide imports, lack of sprayers, absence of vehicles, disorder and confusion in the control services and, finally, the urgency caused by the post-war famine. All in all, these conditions encouraged "the steady advance of the insect in such a favorable climatic environment" (Alfaro Moreno 1951, p. 169)[7].

It is worth noting that the Colorado potato beetle endangered the potato crop, Spain's second most important agricultural product after wheat. From three million metric tons at the beginning of the century, production rose to 4.5 million before the civil war. Approximately 450,000 hectares of land were devoted to potato cultivation in 1940, although production was substantially reduced after the war (*Anuario de Estadística Agraria* 1943, p. 208). Various research centers were set up to develop production, including the Iturrieta experimental farm in the Basque Country, under the direction of agriculturist José María Díaz de Mendivil. His

6 See the works of Clark (2007, 2009), McWilliams (2008) and Fourche (2017).

7 Unless otherwise indicated, translations are by the author.

objective was to research new varieties and distribute new plants to farmers (Díaz de Mendivil 1940).

Although he began this work in the 1930s, Díaz de Mendivil developed his work over the following decades, becoming a notable political figure in the province of Álava and leading several agronomic research projects. He was also appointed to coordinate the activities of engineers in the Basque provinces with the help of local authorities and savings banks. As coordinator of a network of primary and secondary school teachers, he mobilized students in the fight against the Colorado potato beetle. His efforts to find resistant plant varieties and parasitic insects were overtaken by arsenic pesticides as the main means of control. Díaz de Mendivil managed to centralize the purchase of hundreds of tons of lead arsenate in these provinces, as well as other insecticides and spraying equipment, which was subsequently sent to the agriculturists and agricultural unions of the new Franco regime[8].

5.4.1. *The role of agronomists*

Díaz de Mendivil is just one example of the many agronomists who developed a brilliant career, both professionally and politically, under the new Franco regime. This body of state engineers was created in the 19th century but expanded in the first decades of the 20th century with teaching centers, experimental farms, phytopathological stations and provincial agronomic offices. By the end of the 1930s, some 400 agronomists were working in areas such as pest control, seed improvement, farm machinery development, irrigation systems, fertilizer application and other research related to Spanish agriculture (Pan Montojo 2005).

The early years of Franco's regime created new career opportunities for these actors. Although some were affected by the political purge (around 10%, some of whom were forced into exile), most stayed on and contributed, with varying degrees of enthusiasm, to the consolidation of the new regime. This contribution ranged from agricultural research projects to pest control and the regime's new political institutions. Two of the first Ministers of Agriculture in Franco's governments (Carlos Rein and Rafael Cavestany) were agronomists. The head of the department at the time was Manuel Goytia, a prominent member of the Falange (Spain's fascist party), who later became a member of the Spanish Parliament (Pan Montojo and Robledo 2011).

The Franco regime's interest in agriculture is evidenced by the support of political authorities, including the presence of the Head of State at the congress of the Association of Agronomists held in Madrid in 1950 (Congreso 1950).

8 AGA, 61/798. *Pests of the year report* 1945. Álava. January 21, 1946. See also *Agricultura*, 13(1944), p. 152.

This support is also evident in centers such as the Spanish National Research Council (CSIC). These were centers reformed or created in the early months of the new regime, having benefited from the resources and legacy of several institutions that had preceded them (Gomis Blanco 2014).

Like other Francoist engineers, agronomists found new opportunities to develop their modernization projects, with the support of the new regime. These projects used both material products such as pesticides and discourses linked to Franco's ideological universe. As high-ranking civil servants in state institutions with good relations with the political and military authorities, these engineers put their knowledge and networks at the service of the new rulers. Their projects in the fields of agriculture, transport and irrigation also served to legitimize Franco's politics and to frame the affected communities by means of various forms of coercion, either through technocratic planning or through more or less visible symbolic or material violence[9].

The case of the fight against the Colorado potato beetle is a good example of co-production between agrochemical technologies and the Franco dictatorship. On the one hand, and with the help of engineers such as Díaz de Mendivil, programs to disseminate resistant varieties of seed potatoes were stepped up. Delivery took place through new structures in the regime, so that provincial agronomic offices and agricultural unions were responsible for labeling potato seed, providing information on where it could be grown, offering machinery and fertilizers at reduced prices and organizing training courses to teach the new cultivation techniques. On the other hand, with the help of political and military authorities, agronomists were also responsible for punishing reluctant farmers who failed to follow their orders in pest control. Pest control using arsenic sprayers and pesticides was thus presented as a patriotic necessity, in line with the progress and modernization promised by the new dictatorial regime. Moreover, the call to defend the homeland threatened by pests used a whole series of metaphors referring to the war against the Republican groups, i.e. to those who were defeated, exiled or marginalized after the civil war (Pérez Criado and Bertomeu Sánchez 2020).

Pest control services were reformed in August 1940, when a centralized network of agronomists was created. Ranked according to danger and incidence, insects such as locusts and Colorado potato beetles were those that caused the most concern. Locusts were the most persistent insects and were considered the most damaging to Spanish agriculture, with a severe crisis between 1939 and 1940 due to the lack of pesticides, equipment and manpower (Buj 1996).

9 See the study on agronomists (Bertomeu Sánchez 2019b) and on the body of engineers during the Franco dictatorship (Swyngedouw 2015; Camprubí Bueno 2017).

As for the Colorado potato beetle, it was declared a "public disaster" in the summer of 1940. While locusts were visible and their consequences were well known to agriculturists, Colorado potato beetles were difficult to spot and were not perceived as a danger to crops, at least initially. Agronomists urged farmers to inspect their land carefully and report any sign of them as a matter of urgency, even if they saw no danger.

The Potato Sanitary Defense Service (Servicio de Defensa Sanitaria del Cultivo de la Patata) was created the same year, under the supervision of agronomist Agustín Alfaro Moreno. In each province, this service set up increased surveillance to detect new outbreaks, thanks to specially trained staff. It also managed the acquisition of arsenic products and spraying equipment, distributed free or at low cost, with the aim of encouraging future purchases by farmers. Francoist new agricultural unions (Hermandades Sindicales de Labradores y Ganaderos) also distributed lead arsenate at affordable prices (Herráez 2008).

While various methods of controlling the Colorado potato beetle were known at the beginning of the 20th century, arsenic pesticides played a key role in linking the protection of agriculture with the development of the mineral resource industry in northern Spain. On the contrary, the products were expensive, of questionable effectiveness, and made from arsenic, a compound known for its criminal use and the mass poisoning it could cause (Bertomeu Sánchez 2023). It took a multimedia campaign to convince farmers to use them: public lectures, practical courses, brochures, newspaper articles, radio broadcasts and even documentaries.

5.4.2. *Campaigns and resistance: the case of the Burgos province*

To understand the variety of activities carried out by agronomists and their implication in the new regime, as well as the resistance of rural communities, this section is focused on a particular context: the agronomic office of the province of Burgos, a region in central Spain with significant potato production. Eufemio Olmedo Ortega (1891–1954), who was in charge of this office when the Colorado potato beetle arrived, already had over two decades' worth of experience as an agronomist. During the civil war, he held a number of senior positions, including the most senior position on the Commission for Agriculture between 1936 and 1938.

As head of the office, Olmedo visited areas affected by the Colorado potato beetle as early as 1940, the year in which the insect was first detected in fields. He distributed samples of arsenic pesticides and organized conferences on the preparation of arsenic broths. He also published articles in the Diario de Burgos, the most significant Franco regime newspaper in the region. Thanks to his efforts, he obtained the collaboration of the municipal authorities (organizing meetings), the police (the Guardia Civil, which monitored farmland and denounced farmers' inaction) and the political government of the province (with the press publication of financial threats to reluctant farmers)[10].

In Burgos, as in other places, campaigns to distribute arsenic pesticides were greeted with suspicion by some farmers. They were aware of the potential risks of arsenic to their families, livestock and other crops, especially small plots for home consumption and local markets. Indeed, they were more concerned about the lack or excess of rainfall and rising plant prices than about the nuisance of an unknown pest such as the Colorado potato beetle. The first information meetings organized by the mayors did not attract their attention, and only a small group responded to the call, without much enthusiasm[11].

A few farmers did perceive the danger of the new pest, which hardly affected their fields, as its presence was rare and inconspicuous. Others did not report its presence, fearing that their crops would be burnt or that they would not be able to sell their potatoes at the highest price[12]. Faced with this resistance, the political and agricultural authorities imposed heavy fines and financial penalties on reluctant farmers. In the province of Álava, the Provincial Council sent a list of "defaulting farmers" to town halls each year, and also sent personalized letters "informing them of their obligation to comply with all the rules imposed on them"[13].

Eufemio Olmedo also threatened to fine the mayors of municipalities whose fields were affected by the Colorado potato beetle. Manuel Yllera García-Lago, a civilian governor and Franco politician with a history of brutal repression against the anti-fascist resistance, was commissioned to lead the fight against the insect, while coordinating the activities of the Falange for these and other issues. The examples illustrate the extent to which the control of pests and farmers is the result of both political and technological co-production. Indeed, propaganda, agricultural extension and coercion practices were implemented to ensure the submission of rural communities.

The massive use of arsenic pesticides did not, however, prevent the Colorado beetle from becoming endemic in most of the Iberian Peninsula, so pest control treatments had to be repeated every year. The arrival of DDT in 1945 did not mean the end of the arsenic-based pesticides, although it did reduce their consumption until they were later banned.

---

10 AGA, 61/822. Pests of the year report 1941. Eufemio Olmedo. Burgos, December 1942.

11 Burgos Municipal Archives (Archives municipales de Burgos – AMB), 12/1235. Response from the civil authority of the Villatoro district (Burgos), June 14, 1941.

12 AGA, 61/822. Pests of the year report 1941. Eufemio Olmedo. Burgos, December 1942.

13 AGA 61/798. Pests of the year report 1944.

5.5. The arrival of DDT

Organochlorine pesticides arrived in Spain around 1945. Although DDT was synthesized at the end of the 19th century, its properties as a pesticide became known through the research carried out by Paul Müller at the Geigy laboratories in Switzerland, during World War II (Straumann 2005). It was first used in military campaigns by the American army in Italy against typhus and malaria insect vectors. With the support of the Rockefeller Foundation, DDT was adopted in public health and agriculture in many Latin American and European countries in the mid-1940s[14].

Thanks to military and public health campaigns, and the presumed absence of acute toxicity, DDT was presented as the triumph of modern technology over pests and disease. This positive image encouraged its use in urban areas, military barracks, schools, transport vehicles, food establishments and domestic spaces. It also gave rise to a technocratic discourse based on the dream of controlling nature, both insects and diseases (Drouin 2014). Its arrival also encouraged the adoption of other synthetic pesticides and the marginalization of other types of pest control practices, such as biological control (Clarke 2012).

Despite the positive image of these new pesticides, their use was contested by various groups, even though their voices remained unheard for decades. Numerous toxicological studies were carried out shortly after their introduction, providing experimental evidence of the potential danger to mammals. In addition, public health experts urged caution with insecticide-based eradication methods, highlighting the complex interaction between chemicals, insects, disease, humans and the environment. Entomologists and agronomists raised similar points, particularly when they gathered evidence of increasing insect resistance from laboratory studies. Public health or entomology researchers were not the only ones to doubt the safety of the new pesticides; beekeepers and hunters quickly became aware of the damage caused to insects and wildlife in general (Suryanarayanan and Kleinman 2017; Frøyen 2019).

Faced with this reluctance, the chemical industry developed publicity campaigns in the press, radio and television, aimed at dispelling doubts about the benefits of DDT as a non-toxic chemical. These media campaigns, combined with agronomic experiments, silenced studies demonstrating the potential toxicity to mammals of organochlorine pesticides and marginalized calls for precaution (Mart 2015; Conis 2022).

---

14 See the examples of Mexico (Bravo et al. 2020) and Italy (Palmieri 2010). For the Rockefeller Foundation's role, see Stapleton (1998). See also the most recent review by Conis (2022).

In the early 1940s, organochlorine pesticides in Spain were only known in small circles of agronomists and doctors. Alfaro Moreno began laboratory experiments on DDT as early as 1942 and concluded that it had remarkable properties for agricultural use: comparable action to other pesticides on adult insects, and stability in aqueous suspensions facilitating "uniform spraying". He also noted that DDT "did not appear to be toxic to warm-blooded animals at the concentrations commonly used in plant treatment". The main problem was its high price (Alfaro Moreno 1944, pp. 35–36).

Over the following years, Alfaro Moreno continued his field experiments with a dozen commercial preparations of DDT and products based on hexachlorocyclohexane (sometimes called "666"). Some of these were manufactured by Spanish industries under agreements with foreign ones. The production of hexachlorocyclohexane at Cóndor Industries in northwest Spain has been hailed as one of the most significant contributions of early Franco science by contemporary chemists and historians alike[15]. Field studies showed that 666 could be used against the Colorado potato beetle, the difficulty being in the bad taste it gave to potatoes[16], but this problem was quickly solved with the adoption of the lindane isomer (also named "gammaxene"). Despite its known effects on human health, lindane was used in Spain until the 1970s, before becoming one of the main issues of groundwater pollution, which remains unresolved in many areas of Spain (Pérez 2022).

During the summer of 1943, another agronomist, Miguel Benlloch, carried out over a hundred laboratory and field experiments with new organochlorine pesticides (DDT and 666). Benlloch described several advantages of the new products, but criticized excessive optimism about their usefulness and inoffensive nature. In his view, DDT could be ineffective against certain pests and harmful to beneficial insects such as bees. In the absence of sufficient research, he questioned the initial conclusions concerning the absence of toxicity to mammals (Benlloch 1945a, 1945b, 1945c).

Despite the reasonable doubts and known drawbacks of organochlorine insecticides, they became the most widely used products against the Colorado potato beetle in the 1950s. In 1945, in the province of Albacete, agronomists carried out experiments with DDT, obtaining "excellent results" on adult insects and larvae[17]. Trials with organochlorines continued in the years that followed, although the most

15 Two examples from 1940s publications are Gomeza Ozámiz (1945) and Sánchez Buedo (1946). Among current studies celebrating this contribution by Spanish chemists and apothecaries in the early years of Franco's regime, see the work of Andrés Turrión (2019).

16 See, for example, Alfaro Moreno and Alfaro García (1974, pp. 132–134); and Cañizo and González de Andrés (1955, p. 121).

17 AGA, 61/798. Pests of the year report 1945. Albacete, December 31, 1945. Report signed by Miguel Pintado.

purchased products by agronomic offices remained those based on arsenic[18]. By way of comparison, between 1948 and 1949, three tons of lead arsenate and four tons of calcium arsenate were sold in the province of Zamora. This figure dropped to 400 kg for organochlorine insecticides (DDT) in 1948, but significantly increased the following year (1,739 kg)[19].

5.6. Controlling quality, neglecting risk

One of the main concerns of agronomists in the 1940s was pesticide quality control. Indeed, the increase in their demand led to the appearance of poor-quality products, which were sometimes adulterated, altered or were fraudulent versions that caused damage to plants and had no insecticidal effect. The main fear was that these fraudulent products would reinforce farmers' resistance to using pesticides. The engineers argued for the need to establish control measures similar to those existing in other countries and succeeded in bringing about some regulatory advances.

When the pest control service was reformed in 1940, the production and trade of pesticides was placed under the supervision of the agronomic body. Two years later, the Spanish national register of plant protection products was created, almost at the same time as a similar service in Vichy France (Jas 2007). In both cases, the aim was to promote the national pesticide industry and prosecute fraud and adulteration[20].

The pesticide approval process involved a prior report from the provincial agronomic office, sometimes accompanied by additional data on the promoter's other activities, as well as comments on its relationship with Franco's regime. It is highly likely that corruption, nepotism and client networks played an important role in the awarding of contracts, as was the case in other areas, including industrial contamination, water quality or the management of toxic residues (Corral Broto 2018).

Once this initial filter had been passed, the manufacturer would send samples of the pesticides for analysis in the laboratory of the Madrid plant pathology station. Benlloch would then draw up reports on their insecticidal effects, their harmlessness to plants and the possible existence of similar products. He paid particular attention to chemical composition (concentration of active ingredient), physical properties (grain fineness, suspension, solubility, adhesion), persistence in plants, dosage, price

18 AGA, 61/798. Pests of the year report 1947. Albacete, December 31, 1945. Report signed by Miguel Pintado.

19 AGA, 61/1018. Pests of the year report 1949. Zamora, August 1950. Report signed by Francisco Traver.

20 *Boletín Oficial del Estado* (BOE), October 23, 1942.

and means of preparation. Some 900 products were analyzed between 1943 and 1950 (Benlloch 1951).

During the early years, a significant proportion of the products tested (around 28–30%) were rejected and they could not be marketed in Spain. Human toxicity played a very minor role, even in the case of arsenic-based insecticides. The main reasons for rejection were the damage to plants due to its caustic nature and the existence of insecticides that were already manufactured by Spanish industry. Another reason was quality control (composition, efficacy), for which Benlloch carried out a dual chemical and clinical analysis on insects.

However, the arrival of organochlorines created new quality control problems. As Spanish agronomists were familiar with the testing of arsenic-based products, they adapted chemical tests and carried out experimental research to clarify the insecticidal properties of these commercial preparations. They standardized official analytical methods for arsenic products, which were made compulsory by a decree published in 1946. However, methods for testing mixtures of recently synthesized organic isomers proved inadequate. Agronomists and chemists set out in search of new analytical methods (Ruiz Castro 1942, 1947; Hercé 1943, 1945).

These efforts on quality control show a distinction with the weakness of measures taken to avoid risks to farm workers, rural communities and consumers. A number of actors have attempted to make these health and environmental risks visible and to draw the attention of public authorities, but to no avail. These included the press, which relayed the hunters' complaints about the disappearance of rabbits and birds after spraying. The medical profession also called for restrictions on the marketing of pesticides, following several episodes of collective intoxication. Only a few measures have been adopted, particularly to avoid confusion in grocery stores[21].

In this context, no regulations were introduced to control the presence of poisons such as arsenic in food until the 1960s. Aurelio Ruiz Castro, an agronomist that was familiar with the issue, noted that the toxic effects had hardly been studied in the long term. He denounced the excessive number of plant protection products used in Spain, as well as the "unparalleled lightness" of modern agricultural therapeutics, and lamented the lack of information for Spanish consumers, who had no reference works like Rachel Carson's in the United States. His work led to the publication of the first classification of crop protection products, according to their danger to consumers (Ruiz Castro 1966).

The blind spot in this classification remained agricultural workers, subject to chronic, invisible exposure. Indeed, regulations on risk prevention in agricultural

21 *BOE*, December 7, 1946.

work have mostly focused on accidents and physical injuries in 20th-century Spain. Toxicological research in the fields was complex to study, due to the temporality of the workers and their open spaces. It was only in the mid-1960s that agronomists and occupational doctors began to take a real interest in the toxic risks faced by these types of workers (Martínez Linares 1965; Ruiz Castro and Laborda 1965).

5.7. Conclusion

With the help of agronomists and the autarky policies of the new Franco regime, pesticides were massively introduced into Spanish agriculture in the 1940s and presented as the priority means of controlling pests (particularly the Colorado potato beetle). This approach marginalized other methods such as biological control, which was already well developed in the first half of the 20th century. Agricultural research and public action focused on quality and fraud control, while neglecting the production of toxicological and epidemiological data on pesticide poisoning.

Agronomists played a key role in shaping both nature and society in the early days of Franco's dictatorship. Through multimedia campaigns and new regulations, they advocated the use of pesticides as a priority means of combating pest insects, while at the same time developing forms of social control based on the regime's political structures. Pest control also involved rural control through agricultural extension campaigns, which complemented more explicit forms of coercion, such as field incineration, land confiscation, fines and the imprisonment of reluctant farmers.

At the same time, Franco's regime provided an ideal framework for the development of agronomic modernization projects and the pesticide industry. The introduction of arsenic pesticides paved the way for organochlorine products, which were presented as harmless. Chronic, invisible exposure was ignored, despite early warnings of the risks to workers, consumers and the environment. There was a stark contrast between public inaction in the face of these risks, and the resources invested in researching the effects of pesticides on insects and plants.

The fight against the Colorado potato beetle was carried out at the same time as the violent repression of anti-fascist resistance. Brandishing arsenic pesticides, agronomists and political authorities were able to present themselves as Spain's protectors against the Colorado potato beetle invasion, often using terms similar to the fight against subversive groups.

5.8. References

Alfaro Moreno, A. (1944). *La lucha química contra el escarabajo de la patata en España*. Dirección General de Agricultura, Madrid.

Alfaro Moreno, A. (1945). *Una calamidad pública: La plaga del escarabajo de la patata*. Dirección General de Agricultura, Madrid.

Alfaro Moreno, A. (1947). La eficacia de los insecticidas agrícolas a base de DDT y 666 en la lucha contra el escarabajo de la patata. *Boletín de Patología Vegetal y Entomología Agrícola*, 15, 175–193.

Alfaro Moreno, A. (1951). La invasión del escarabajo de la patata y problemas planteados. *Boletín de Patología Vegetal y Entomología Agrícola*, 18, 139–177.

Alfaro Moreno, A. and Alfaro García, A. (1974). *Plaguicidas agrícolas*. Inia, Madrid.

Andrés Turrión, M.L. (2019). La compañía Insecticidas Cóndor S. A. y el desarrollo del hexa-cloro-benceno en la posguerra española. In *Ciencia útil: Investigación básica y aplicada en Farmacia y Ciencias de la Vida*, González Bueno, A. and Baratas Díaz, A. (eds). Ediciones Complutense, Madrid, 181–208.

Aportaciones (1944). Aportaciones del Estado en la lucha contra el escarabajo de la patata. *Agricultura*, 13(142), 88–92.

Arancibia, F. and Motta, R. (2019). Undone science and counter-expertise: Fighting for justice in an Argentine community contaminated by pesticides. *Science as Culture*, 28(3), 277–302.

Bellod, M. (1957). Análisis de insecticidas mixtos de DDT y lindano. *Boletín de Patología Vegetal y Entomología Agrícola*, 25, 273–290.

Benlloch, M. (1945a). Ensayos de laboratorio sobre la acción por contacto de los insecticidas orgánicos clorados (DDT y 666). *Boletín de Patología Vegetal y Entomología Agrícola*, 14, 189–198.

Benlloch, M. (1945b). Los nuevos insecticidas orgánicos. *Agricultura*, 14(162), 511–516.

Benlloch, M. (1945c). Observaciones sobre la eficacia insecticida de los preparados a base de DDT y gama-hexano. *Boletín de Patología Vegetal y Entomología Agrícola*, 14, 343–352.

Benlloch, M. (1951). El servicio de comprobación y registro de productos fitoterapéuticos. *Boletín de Patología Vegetal y Entomología Agrícola*, 18, 123–129.

Bertomeu Sánchez, J.R. (2019a). Pesticides, past and present. A review of current literature. *HoST – Journal of History of Science and Technology*, 13(1), 1–27.

Bertomeu Sánchez, J.R. (2019b). Arsenical pesticides in early Francoist Spain: Fascism, autarky, agricultural engineers and the invisibility of toxic risks. *HoST – Journal of History of Science and Technology*, 13(1), 53–82.

Bertomeu Sánchez, J.R. (2020a). El escarabajo del Marqués. Violencia lenta, plaguicidas arsenicales y cine agrario durante los primeros años del franquismo. In *Tóxicos Invisibles. La construcción de la ignorancia ambiental*, Guillem, X. and Nieto, A. (eds). Icaria, Barcelona, 79–109.

Bertomeu Sánchez, J.R. (2020b). Poisons in the twentieth century: Unpunished crimes, slow violence and the role of history. *Cahiers François Viète*, 9, 105–122.

Bertomeu Sánchez, J.R. (2021). *Tóxicos: pasado y presente. Pensar históricamente un mundo tóxico*. Icaria, Barcelona.

Boudia, S. and Henry, E. (2022). *Politiques de l'ignorance*. PUF, Paris.

Boudia, S., Creager, A.N.H., Frickel, S., Henry, E., Jas, N., Reinhardt, C., Roberts, J.A. (2021). *Residues: Thinking Through Chemical Environments*. Rutgers University Press, New Brunswick.

Boutelou Soldevilla, E. (1877). La Dorífora, escarabajo del Colorado o de la patata. *Gaceta agrícola del Ministerio de Fomento*, 5, 63–66.

Bravo, S.F., Bertomeu Sánchez, J.R., Aceves, L.S. (2020). Adopción y producción estatal de DDT en México (1940–1980). *Estudios de Historia Moderna y Contemporánea de México*, 60, 257–292.

Buj, A. (1996). *La lucha contra la langosta en la España contemporánea*. Ministerio de Agricultura, Alimentación y Medio Ambiente, Madrid.

Camprubí Bueno, L. (2017). *Los ingenieros de Franco*. Editorial Crítica, Barcelona.

Cañizo, J. (1928). Una amenaza para el cultivo de la patata: El escarabajo de la patata. *Boletín de Patología Vegetal y Entomología Agrícola*, 3, 36–41.

Cañizo, J. (1932). La Dorífora de la patata en Francia. Grave peligro para nuestra agricultura. *Agricultura*, 44, 495–497.

Cañizo, J. and González de Andrés, C. (1955). *Manual práctico de fitopatología y terapéutica agrícola*. Ministerio de Agricultura, Madrid.

Cano Manuel, J.R. (1979). Evolución del consumo de fitosanitarios en España. *Boletín del Servicio de Plagas*, 5, 203–213.

Clark, J.F.M. (2007). "The eyes of our potatoes are weeping": The rise of the Colorado beetle as an insect pest. *Archives of Natural History*, 34, 109–128.

Clark, J.F.M. (2009). *Bugs and the Victorians*. Yale University Press, New Haven.

Clarke, S. (2012). Rethinking the post war hegemony of DDT. In *Environment, Health and History*, Berridge, V. and Gorksky, M. (eds). Palgrave Macmillan, New York, 133–153.

Clarke, S. and Lean, T. (2022). Turning DDT into 'Didimac': Making insecticide products and consumers in British farming after 1945. *History and Technology*, 38, 1–31.

Congreso (1950). *Congreso Nacional de Ingeniería Agronómica*. Asociación Nacional de Ingenieros Agronómos, Madrid.

Conis, E. (2022). *How to Sell a Poison: The Rise, Fall, and Toxic Return of DDT*. Bold Type Books, New York.

Corral Broto, P. (2018). Historia de la corrupción ambiental en España, 1939-1979. ¿Franquismo o industrialización? *Hispania Nova*, 33, 646–684.

Davis, F.R. (2019). Pesticides and the perils of synecdoche in the history of science and environmental history. *History of Science*, 57(4), 469–492.

Dedieu, F., Jouzel, J.-N., Prete, G. (2015). Governing by ignoring. The production and the function of the under-reporting of farm-workers' pesticide poisoning in French and Californian regulations. In *Handbook of Ignorance Studies*, Gross, M. and McGoey, L. (eds). Routledge, London, 297–307.

Díaz de Mendivil, J.M. (1940). Las variedades de patata y su influencia en el cultivo. *Agricultura*, 96(124), 139–144.

Dirección General de Agricultura (1953). *Plagas del campo. VI. Registro de Productos y Material Fitosanitario*. Ministerio de Agricultura, Madrid.

Drouin, J.-M. (2014). *Philosophie de l'insecte*. Le Seuil, Paris.

Fernández Prieto, L., Pan Montojo, J., Cabo, M. (eds) (2014). *Agriculture in the Age of Fascism: Authoritarian Technocracy and Rural Modernization, 1922–1945*. Brepols, Brussels.

Fitzgerald, D. (2010). *Every Farm a Factory. The Industrial Ideal in American Agriculture*. Yale University Press, New Haven.

Fourche, R. (2004). Contribution à l'histoire de la protection phytosanitaire dans l'agriculture française (1880-1970). PhD Thesis, Université Lyon 2, Lyon.

Fourche, R. (2017). Internationalisation des traitements arsenicaux : des doryphores américains aux abeilles françaises (1868–1922). *Histoire & Sociétés Rurales*, 47(2), 137–176.

Frøyen, A.J. (2019). Influencing for results: Bees, beekeepers and Norwegian Pesticide Legislation. *HoST – Journal of History of Science and Technology*, 13(1), 28–50.

Gomeza Ozámiz, J.M. (1945). El descubrimiento del nuevo insecticida 666. *Ión*, 5(53), 745–750.

Gomis Blanco, A. (2014). Mimbres para otro cesto: De la Sección de Entomología del Museo Nacional de Ciencias Naturales al Instituto Español de Entomología. *Boletín de la Real Sociedad Española de Historia Natural*, 108(1–4), 37–47.

González de Molina, M., Soto Fernández, D., Guzmán Casado, G. (2020). *The Social Metabolism of Spanish Agriculture, 1900–2008*. Springer Open, Cham.

Guillem Llobat, X. (2019). Following hydrogen cyanide in the Valencian Country (1907–1933): Risk, accidents and standards in fumigation. *HoST – Journal of History of Science and Technology*, 13(1), 51–75.

Guthman, J. (2019). *Wilted. Pathogens, Chemicals, and the Fragile Future of the Strawberry Industry*. University of California Press, Berkeley.

Hercé, P. (1943). *Condiciones que deben exigirse a los insecticidas arsenicales*. Ministerio de Agricultura, Madrid.

Hercé, P. (1945). *Análisis de insecticidas*. Instituto Nacional de Investigaciones Agronómicas, Madrid.

Herráez, J.M.G. (2008). Las hermandades sindicales de labradores y ganaderos (1942–1977): Del análisis franquista a la historiografía actual. *Historia Agraria*, 44, 119–155.

Jansen, S. (2000). Chemical-warfare techniques for insect control: Insect “pests” in Germany before and after World War I. *Endeavour*, 24(1), 28–33.

Jas, N. (2005). Déqualifier le paysan, introniser l’agronome, Allemagne 1840–1914. *Écologie et politique*, 31(2), 45–55.

Jas, N. (2007). Public health and pesticide regulation in France before and after Silent Spring. *History and Technology*, 23(4), 369–388.

Jas, N. (2011). *Au carrefour de la chimie et de l’agriculture: les sciences agronomiques en Allemagne et en Allemagne, 1850-1914*. Editions des archives contemporaines, Paris.

Jasanoff, S. (ed.). (2004). *States of Knowledge. The Co-Production of Science and Social Order*. Routledge, London.

Jouzel, J.N. (2019). *Pesticides. Comment ignorer ce que l’on sait*. Presses de Sciences Po, Paris.

Kourany, J. and Carrier, M. (2020). *Science and the Production of Ignorance: When the Quest for Knowledge Is Thwarted*. MIT, Cambridge.

Lyons, K. (2018). Chemical warfare in Colombia, evidentiary ecologies and senti-actuando practices of justice. *Social Studies of Science*, 48(3), 414–437.

Lyons, K. (2020). *Vital Decomposition: Soil Practitioners & Life Politics*. Duke University Press, Durham.

Mart, M. (2015). *Pesticides, a Love Story: America’s Enduring Embrace of Dangerous Chemicals*. University Press of Kansas, Lawrence.

Martínez Linares, V. (1965). Acción tóxica de los plaguicidas y reacción orgánica frente a la agresión de estos productos. *Revista de Medicina y Seguridad en el Trabajo*, 51, 46–57.

McWilliams, J.E. (2008). *American Pests: The Losing War on Insects from Colonial Times to DDT*. Columbia University Press, New York.

Murray, D.L. (1994). *Cultivating Crisis: The Human Cost of Pesticides in Latin America*, 3rd edition. University of Texas Press, Austin.

Nagore, D. (1939). *La patata: El tubérculo de los incas*. Aramburu, Pamplona.

Nieto Galan, A. (2019). *The Politics of Chemistry. Science and Power in 20th-Century Spain*. Cambridge University Press, Cambridge.

Palmieri, W. (2010). Environmental imperialism in Sardinia: Pesticides and politics in the struggle against malaria. In *Nature and History in Modern Italy*, Armiero, M. and Hall, M. (eds). Ohio University Press, Athens.

Pan Montojo, J. (2005). *Apostolado, profesión y tecnología: una historia de los ingenieros agrónomos en España*. Asociación Nacional de Ingenieros Agrónomos, Madrid.

Pan Montojo, J. and Robledo, R. (eds) (2011). *Historia del Ministerio de Agricultura, 1900 2008: Política agraria y pesquera de España*. Ministerio de Medio Ambiente y Medio Rural y Marino, Centro de Publicaciones, Madrid.

Pérez, O.A. (2022). Un plaguicida en el franquismo: Comunicación de riesgos tóxicos en España, 1945-1975. *História, Ciências, Saúde – Manguinhos*, 29(2), 421–440.

Pérez Criado, S. (2017). El legado de Rachel Carson. *Anales de Química*, 113(4), 88–96.

Pérez Criado, S. and Bertomeu Sánchez, J.R. (2020). From arsenic to DDT: Making invisible the risks of pesticides in the early years of Francoist Spain (1939–1953). *Cultural & History Journal*, 10(1). doi: 10.3989/chdj.2021.004.

Phillips, J. and French, M. (1998). The pure beer campaign and arsenic poisoning, 1896–1903. *Rural History: Economy, Society, Culture*, 9, 195–209.

Proctor, R. and Schiebinger, L. (eds) (2008). *Agnotology: The Making and Unmaking of Ignorance*. Stanford University Press, Redwood City.

Quintana Marí, A. (1944). Contribución al estudio físico-químico del β β β-Tricloro-αα bis (p. clorofenil)-etano y su determinación analítica en los insecticidas preparados a base del mismo. *Boletín de Patología Vegetal y Entomología Agrícola*, 13, 229–270.

Quintana Marí, A. and Cid Capella, A.M. (1946). Una nueva reacción colorimétrica del DDT. *Boletín del Instituto Nacional de Investigaciones Agronómicas*, 15, 118–221.

Riegert, P.W. (1980). *From Arsenic to DDT: A History of Entomology in Western Canada*. University of Toronto Press, Toronto.

Romero, A.M. (2021). *Economic Poisoning: Industrial Waste and the Chemicalization of American Agriculture*. University of California Press, Berkeley.

Ruiz Castro, A. (1942). Algunos casos dudosos en el análisis de insecticidas arsenicales. *Boletín de Patología Vegetal y Entomología Agrícola*, 11, 331–38.

Ruiz Castro, A. (1947). Algunas posibles sofisticaciones de los insecticidas arsenicales. *Boletín de Patología Vegetal y Entomología Agrícola*, 15, 194–222.

Ruiz Castro, A. (1958). Métodos de análisis de productos fitoterapéuticos. I. Dicloro-Difenil-Tricloroetano. *Boletín de Patología Vegetal y Entomología Agrícola*, 25, 231–249.

Ruiz Castro, A. (1966). Plaguicidas Agrícolas: Toxicidad Residual y Salud Pública. *Boletín de Patología Vegetal y Entomología Agrícola*, 29, 1–32.

Ruiz Castro, A. and Laborda, E. (1965). Principales productos fitosanitarios utilizados en España y tipo de formulaciones de aplicación agrícola. *Revista de Medicina y Seguridad en el Trabajo*, 51, 8–18.

Russell, E. (2001). *War and Nature: Fighting Humans and Insects with Chemicals from World War I to Silent Spring*. Cambridge University Press, Cambridge.

Sánchez Buedo, E. (1946). Un nuevo insecticida orgánico. El hexaclorociclоexano (666) y su isómero más activo, el gamma (gammexane). *Agricultura*, 15(167), 124–127.

Saraiva, T. (2016). *Fascist Pigs: Technoscientific Organisms and the History of Fascism*. MIT Press, Cambridge.

Spear, R.J. (2005). *The Great Gypsy Moth War*. University of Massachusetts Press, Amherst.

Stapleton, D.H. (1998). The dawn of DDT and its experimental use by the Rockefeller Foundation in Mexico, 1943–1952. *Parassitologia*, 40, 149–158.

Straumann, L. (2005). *Nützliche Schädlinge: Angewandte Entomologie, chemische Industrie und Landwirtschaftspolitik in der Schweiz 1874–1952*. Chronos, Zurich.

Suay Matallana, I. and Guillem Llobat, X. (2018). Poisoned wine: Regulation, chemical analyses, and Spanish-French Trade in the 1930s. *Ambix*, 1–23.

Suryanarayanan, S. and Kleinman, D.L. (2017). *Vanishing Bees: Science, Politics, and Honeybee Health*. Rutgers University Press, New Brunswick.

Swyngedouw, E. (2015). *Liquid Power: Contested Hydro-Modernities in Twentieth-Century Spain*. MIT Press, Cambridge.

Whorton, J. (1974). *Before Silent Spring: Pesticides and Public Health in Pre-DDT America*. Princeton University Press, Princeton.

Wright, A. (2005). *The Death of Ramón González: The Modern Agricultural Dilemma*. University of Texas Press, Austin.

6

From Pesticides to Thyroid Diseases: Media Coverage of a Nameless Problem

6.1. Introduction

As a result of an ongoing research project (ThyroSIC), aiming to analyze and understand the publicization of thyroid diseases in France, as well as their inclusion within the national public health policies, this work specifically focuses on the media coverage of the links between pesticides and thyroid diseases. For many years, a growing number of scientific studies have demonstrated etiological links between pesticides' use and various health problems, linked, for example, to growth and reproduction. More recently, new studies have also shown impacts on the thyroid gland functioning. Indeed, scientific studies show links between the use of certain pesticides and increased thyroid dysfunction, through a number of endocrine disruptors. This is notably the case demonstrated in the literature review carried out by Erbs and Joubert (2017), or that of Michel Pugeat, whose work highlights the need to apply the precautionary principle to maternal and child exposure to pollutants, because of the relationships between such exposure and certain thyroid gland pathologies (Pugeat 2017).

On the other side of the Atlantic, studies by Whitney S. Goldner demonstrated a 12% increase in cases of hypothyroidism in the pesticide-exposed population, compared to the general population. More specifically, this study demonstrated links between the onset of hypothyroidism and women's exposure to certain organochlorine insecticides and fungicides (Goldner et al. 2010). In terms of public actors and work carried out by European institutions, a 2013 report by the EFSA (European Food Safety Authority), aimed to identify pesticides to include within the

---

Chapter written by Estera BADAU.

cumulative assessment groups on the basis of their toxicological profile, shows that, out of 287 substances assessed, 101 were identified as affecting the thyroid or the thyroid hormones (EFSA 2013).

In France, for some years now, associations such as *Alerte des médecins sur les pesticides* (AMLP) and *Générations Futures* have been carrying out specific actions and works aimed at questioning French and European public authorities, particularly on the subject of pesticides and endocrine disruptors impacting the functioning of the thyroid gland and the hormones it produces. In 2017 and 2018, for example, the two associations played an active role in discussions in Brussels, with the objective of adopting scientific criteria for determining which endocrine disruptors should be excluded, in compliance with the European regulations on active substances in agricultural pesticides and biocides. In 2021, the two associations jointly published two reports to draw the attention of European public authorities to the need for regulatory change, following the debates of 2017 and 2018. The two associations highlight the European Commission's objectives, which include enabling the exclusion from the market of substances, which may have endocrine-disrupting effects. However, they criticize the approach and explain that the criteria for identifying endocrine disruptors for biocidal active substances and for pesticides, adopted by the European Commission following the 2017 and 2018 debates, are limited by including only two of the three categories of existing endocrine disruptors:

> The assessment criteria adopted in 2017 by the EU after nine years of waiting require a very high level of evidence, retaining only "known" and "alleged" endocrine disruptors. There is no category identifying "suspected" disruptors, unlike mutagenic and reprotoxic carcinogens (CMRs). In other words, those for which not all the evidence has been gathered (Générations Futures 2022).

Therefore, the two reports produced by the above-mentioned associations highlight the concrete changes brought by the adoption of these criteria for 13 active substances, all having three elements in common: they disrupt the functioning of the thyroid gland or its hormones; their marketing authorizations were due to expire in 2021 and they are present in food according to the work of ANSES (2014). The conclusions of both reports point out the shortcomings in the existing regulations and highlight the scientific difficulties of definitively proving etiological links. As a result, the associations' demands mainly call for the adoption of a category of "suspected" endocrine disruptors, as well as a review of the process of automatic extension of approvals.

The main aim of this study is to analyze the media coverage of the links between pesticides and thyroid dysfunction in order to highlight the issues involved in publicizing the subject. To do this, it is helpful to explain the context in which this work was carried out. It stems from an ongoing research project, ThyroSIC, developed within the CIMEOS laboratory works, which focuses on the publicization of thyroid diseases, their mediatization and their inclusion in public health policies. This chapter begins by presenting the theoretical analysis framework (section 6.1). The latter is part of the current body of work on the publicization and media coverage of public problems. A review of the work carried out in the humanities and social sciences on thyroid diseases is then presented (section 6.2). The methodological section (section 6.3) reviews the work involved in building the corpus under analysis (a written press corpus of articles published by the newspaper *Le Monde* from 2000 to 2020) and the analysis method (Robert Entman's theory of framing). Following the pragmatist approach of public problems, the analysis therefore uses tools derived from the work of Robert Entman, highlighting the functions of framing operations and cross-referencing them with the work of Joseph Gusfield. Therefore, while numerous actors and/or groups take ownership of a problem, the definition of its causes and the solutions to be implemented, tensions can emerge between the actors involved in the process of publicizing the issue. The results underline the difficulty of establishing the issue of endocrine-disrupting pesticides and thyroid dysfunction as a public problem, even though this is certainly a public health issue. The analysis of the media coverage of this issue over the last 20 years shows the difficulty of naming the problem, beyond the questions related to its visibility in the public arena and the media agenda, or the difficulties of regulation, in the context of denunciations of conflicts of interest within European public authorities.

6.2. Thyroid diseases: publicization and media coverage

In line with the works developed within the pragmatist approach of public problems (Arquembourg 2016a, 2016b; Cefaï 2016; Badau 2019), the contextual elements briefly presented above enable us to observe several aspects of the publicization (Pailliart 2005) of the links between pesticides and thyroid dysfunction. Firstly, there is the question of multiple actors taking charge of the issue and disputing, what Joseph Gusfield's work would call: the problem ownership, the definition of its causal responsibility and the definition of its political responsibility (Gusfield 1981, 1996). In other words, groups of actors feel they have a right (or are entitled), as owners of the issue, to name and define the problem, identify its causes and designate the actors held responsible for implementing solutions (Badau et al. 2022). From the scientific community to the health and political actors, including the associations and industrialists who take ownership of the problem, the issue to be defended differs and reveals possible confrontations between these different actors.

These confrontations contribute to the production of knowledge and understanding and also lead to the emergence of controversies. Another issue that emerges in this process of publicization is specifically linked to the logic of making the issue (in)visible (Voirol 2005) in the public sphere. The pattern of the publicization process showing the takeover of scientific studies by associative structures, so as to challenge and confront political and health actors (Badau 2019), is neither new nor specific to the issue of pesticides; however, the question of the invisibility and intangibility of the long-term consequences seems to be predominant from the outset in this process of thyroid diseases publicization. As Ulrich Beck states,

> It often happens that what affects health or destroys nature is not identifiable by perception or sight; and even in cases where everything seems obvious, the social construct dictates that we must resort to the "objective" findings of expert judgment (Beck 2008).

The difficulty of proving the links between endocrine-disrupting pesticides and thyroid dysfunction is also present here. If awareness is to be raised, there is a need of scientific expertise and studies on the issue, as well as a need for publicizing this knowledge and these results. Media coverage is one of the ways in which an issue of public interest is publicized and awareness is raised. The media in general, and the written press in particular, play a significant role in the process of publicizing and constituting a public issue. As a "scene of appearance, where successive snapshots of the configuration of a social problem are printed, where the actors who have access to it and the authoritative discourses are made visible and audible" (Arquembourg 2016a, 2016b), the written press offers the possibility of working on a long-term corpus. Beyond the possibility of tracking down some of the actors and groups taking ownership of the problem, as well as their discourses, there is also the question of media coverage and articles framing according to editorial lines, questions linked to layout, article construction, the arrangement of elements making up articles, possible stances, etc. As Jocelyne Arquembourg mentions with regard to the problem of antibiotic resistance, the written press is:

> [A] place that bears traces of the scenes in which actors intervene, in which their statements are exchanged; a place […] that gives a glimpse of the multiplicity of protagonists in these intrigues and the fault lines explaining, in part, why the problem could never be configured, as such, as a unified problem (Arquembourg 2016a, 2016b).

With the aim of analyzing the media coverage of links between pesticides and thyroid dysfunction, this work is based on the analysis of a corpus of written press articles, published by the newspaper *Le Monde* from 2000 to 2020. Rooted in information and communication sciences, and following the pragmatist approach of public problems, the analysis also uses concepts and analytical tools from discourse analysis. Robert Entman's work highlights the functions of framing operations: diagnosis, assessment, recommendation and solution. We therefore consider that it would be interesting to apply this cross-analysis grid between the contributions of Robert Entman and those of Joseph Gusfield, which highlight the existence of multiple definitions of the problem, its causes and its solutions, following the numerous actors and/or groups who take ownership of a problem.

In short, following a diachronic perspective, this study analyzes the articles published in the newspaper *Le Monde* over the last 20 years on the subject of pesticides, endocrine disruptors and thyroid dysfunction, focusing, in particular, on the discursive framings that emerge, as well as the arguments that result from the media coverage and the actors taking ownership of this problem.

6.2.1. *Perspectives from humanities and social sciences research on thyroid diseases*

To date, the matter of thyroid diseases has not been the central focus of research in the humanities and social sciences. Indeed, many works by historians (Boudia and Jas 2019), sociologists (Pena-Vega 2002; Ackerman et al. 2006; Chateauraynaud 2014), psychologists (Orsini 2004; Fischer and Tarquinio 2014) or researchers in information and communication sciences (Moreau 2019; Huet 2020) deal with thyroid diseases in an underlying or marginal way. The latter are often associated with work on cancer, in connection with the debate on nuclear and radioactivity, or on endocrine disruptors and pesticides. More broadly, the analyses provided by these works follow a sociological perspective on risk and warning or on psychosocial aspects. As for work on pesticides and endocrine disruptors, while thyroid disease is sometimes mentioned, there is a lack of in-depth analysis and understanding. To our knowledge, no research work to date in social sciences has investigated thyroid diseases as a central topic.

Thyroid diseases therefore not only suffer from a lack of visibility in the public sphere, but also from a lack of research work analyzing, from a cross-disciplinary perspective, the various ramifications of the problem, the way it is handled by public health actors and the reconfigurations brought about by digital technology. The ThyroSIC project run within the CIMEOS laboratory works at the University of Burgundy addresses these issues, with the aim of considering connections between all of the fields which this issue may affect: health, food and the environment.

6.3. Methodology

6.3.1. *Analytical corpus and methodological aspects*

As a reference newspaper, with an average daily circulation of 452,869 copies in 2021 according to ACPM[1] figures, *Le Monde* is top of the list in the French daily press circulation rankings, while claiming an unbiased and non-partisan approach. Its interest, as a source for the constitution of the corpus, is also linked to the journal functioning and the progressive specialization that the newspaper has implemented, with the creation of specific sections on health or environment, etc.

To build up the analysis corpus, we carried out keyword searches in the Europresse database. An initial search using the root of the keyword "thyroid*" (TEXT = thyroid* → 360)[2] produced a so-called "reference" corpus (Moirand 2007), comprising the 360 articles published by *Le Monde* on the subject of thyroid disease. As Sophie Moirand explains, a reference corpus represents "the global context of the analysis and functions as an analytical reference on which the interpretation of the results is based" (Moirand 2007). This first corpus highlighted peaks in media coverage that either reflect "discursive moments" or "discursive instants" (Moirand 2007), as the histogram in Figure 6.1 shows.

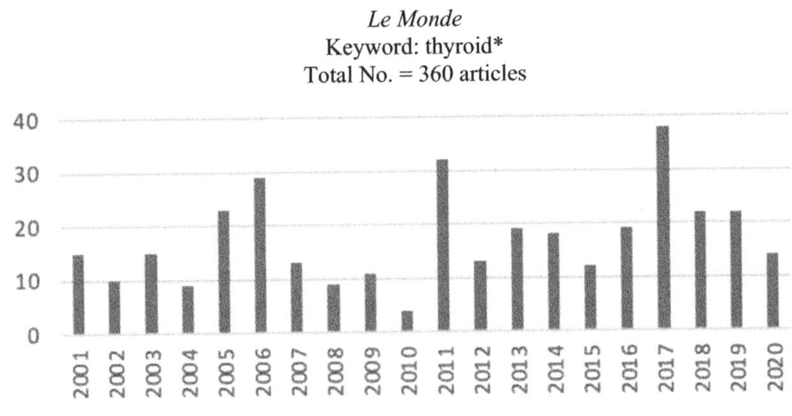

Figure 6.1. *Media coverage of thyroid disease by Le Monde*

1 L'Alliance pour les chiffres de la presse et des médias, ACPM (2022). Classement diffusion presse quotidienne nationale [Online]. Available at: http://www.acpm.fr/Les-chiffres/Diffusion-Presse/Presse-Payante/Presse-Quotidienne-Nationale [Accessed February 21, 2022].

2 The asterisk is used to group together all articles containing the phrase "thyroid". It is particularly useful for finding all articles on thyroid diseases, with the different variations of the word "thyroid", "thyroidal", " hypothyroidism", etc.

While the focus is on the ways in which thyroid-related illnesses come to the forefront during these media peaks, the articles also cover a wide range of thyroid-related issues and reflect a number of controversies surrounding thyroid diseases. The first controversy is linked to nuclear accidents and radioactivity, in connection with the increase in cases of thyroid cancer and the actions taken by patient associations in the form of denunciations, petitions and the questioning of public authorities. From the Chernobyl disaster and its aftermath, to the Fukushima accident in 2011, the issue recurs regularly in articles published by the newspaper *Le Monde* and reflects the confrontations between the protagonists involved (patients, associations, health professionals, public authorities). A second controversial subject on thyroid diseases which has a high profile in the media is the Levothyrox "crisis" in 2017, linked to the change in formula of this drug marketed by Merck. Articles are also gradually reporting on the first ramification of this health problem toward food and nutrition. Indeed, nutritional advice, recommendations and opinions are beginning to circulate, speaking about certain "diets" to be followed by patients suffering from hypothyroid-type dysfunction. Finally, another controversial topic to have emerged in recent years relates to the use of certain pesticides and endocrine disruptors.

While this initial thematic analysis has shown that thyroid diseases have been covered by *Le Monde* over the last 20 years in a variety of ways, it has also highlighted the fact that thyroid disease is linked to the health–food–environment triad. This highlights the need for a cross-disciplinary approach to the study of thyroid diseases.

This first corpus also reveals the existence of journalistic articles dealing with the links between endocrine-disrupting pesticides and certain thyroid dysfunctions.

A second search focused on the media coverage of issues related to pesticides and endocrine disruptors (pesticide* & (endocrine* disruptor*) → 244) brings together articles featuring all three terms or variations thereof. In order to refine the search and find articles which specifically deal with thyroid diseases and endocrine disrupting pesticides, we carried out two further searches (pesticide* & thyroid* → 37 and thyroid* & (endocrine* disruptor*) → 35). The number of articles is smaller. Therefore, the "working" corpus (Moirand 2007) on which the analysis of the present study is based, comprises 37 articles. As the graph in Figure 6.2 shows, the media coverage of the subject in question is very low, and also very recent, with the few articles published by the journal being concentrated around the last few years.

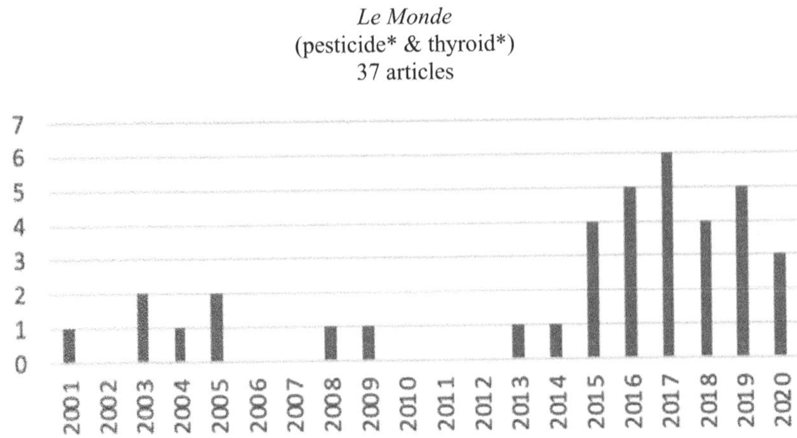

Figure 6.2. *Media coverage of the links between thyroid diseases and endocrine disrupting pesticides by Le Monde*

6.3.2. *Analysis method*

Our approach is based on a semantic–pragmatic perspective of discourse analysis, at the crossroads of various concepts and analytical tools derived from research in information and communication sciences and discourse analysis, where discourse is considered a "set of strategies by a subject, the product of which is a construction characterized by the actors, objects, properties and events on which it operates" (Maingueneau 1987, p. 18). We are thus following the frame-analysis perspective proposed by Robert Entman, who highlights the three functions of framing: diagnosing, evaluating or prescribing a recommendation or solution. As he explains, framing means putting an issue into discourse in such a way as to designate a certain definition of the question, a causal interpretation, a moral assessment and/or a treatment recommendation for the question presented. As the author explains,

> To frame is to select certain aspects of a perceived reality and make them more salient in a communication text, so as to promote a particular problem definition, causal interpretation, moral assessment and/or treatment recommendation for the item described (Entman 1993, p. 51).

Combined with the study of public problems, this perspective makes it possible to work on the definitions that are proposed for a problem by the numerous groups of actors who claim to legitimately tackle the problem. This is also the case regarding the problem of endocrine-disrupting thyroid pesticides, since the media coverage of the subject reflects the plurality of actors involved in the problem: the scientific community, associations and non-governmental organizations (NGOs), international and European public institutions, and industrialists.

6.4. Results: thyroid-disrupting pesticides, a nameless public health problem

While the links between endocrine-disrupting pesticides and thyroid dysfunction have so far received little media coverage in the daily newspapers analyzed, a first salient feature of this media coverage reveals two distinct periods. Before 2013, a dozen articles on a wide variety of subjects mentioned pesticides, most often in connection with the increase in cancer cases. Thyroid cancer is cited in a long list of cancers (lymphoma, multiple myeloma, leukemia, gastrointestinal cancer, kidney cancer, prostate cancer and thyroid cancer). In terms of discursive framing, what emerges as the common thread of the causes of the problem is the environment in the broadest sense (ranging from pesticide use to lifestyles, and including air pollution, occupational but also domestic exposure or recalling the aftermath of the Chernobyl disaster). The specialized term (the absence or inadequacy of "data quantifying exposure and specifying co-exposures"), combined with the fact that most of these articles are published in specialized sections (environment, science, planet), are some of the factors that may explain why the issue is confined to a specific field and aimed at an expert reader, accustomed to scientific work or able to do extra work to understand the subject. However, until now, endocrine disruptors have not really been part of the subject. It was only after 2013 that associations between the latter and thyroid dysfunctions began to receive a certain amount of attention and media coverage. Indeed, in a context of multiplying and increasingly sophisticated scientific studies, followed by actions aimed at implementing regulations at the European Union level, potential links between endocrine-disrupting pesticides and thyroid dysfunctions began to be the subject of journalistic articles.

6.4.1. *From the difficulty of naming reality...*

One of the key elements in the process of publicizing a problem is its name. Indeed, one of the specific features of the pragmatist approach of public problems is the importance given to discourse, and the interest in studying the meanings and implications arising from the ways in which the problem and its solutions are defined and named. Discursive operations are an integral part of the process by which public problems are constituted, enabling us to understand the links which are woven between the definition of a problem and its solutions. As Daniel Cefaï points out, "naming and narrating is already acting, entering into a logic of designation and description of the problem with a view to solving it" (Cefaï 1996, pp. 49–50). Jocelyne Arquembourg's work has demonstrated the value of studying the meanings and implications that come from the ways in which a problem and its solutions are defined. Crossing pragmatist perspectives on the constitution of public problems with Georges Kleiber's work on denominations and designations, the author emphasizes that naming makes it possible to associate an identity with a problem. As she puts it:

> Naming has two functions. It helps to objectify what it designates, so that it exists beyond a point of view. [...] Naming also has the effect of totalizing what it designates under a description. This phenomenon of totalization plays a cognitive role and enables us to understand what we are referring to, as well as endowing it with an identity (Arquembourg 2016a, pp. 29–47).

This is not the case for the problem of linking endocrine-disrupting pesticides and thyroid dysfunction. We do not have a name summing up the elements of this problem, even though scientific knowledge on the matter is growing. For example, as early as 2012, a report by the World Health Organization (WHO) and the United Nations Environment Programme (UNEP) pointed out that "nearly 800 environmental chemicals are known or suspected to interfere with hormone receptors, hormone synthesis or hormone conversion" (Foucart and Santi 2015). Although this second period of media coverage reflects the complexity of the problem, the angle through which the issue of thyroid-disrupting pesticides is beginning to be publicized refers to the numerous future consequences of endocrine disruptors (different types of cancers and also other health problems) and the need to update regulation, taking the scientific literature into account.

Indeed, this second phase of media coverage began in 2013 with an event known as the "Berlaymont Declaration on endocrine disruptors". The declaration represented a motion drafted by scientists from a variety of disciplines, calling on the European Commission to review the regulations governing the use of a number of substances. Stemming from a scientific event held the previous year, the motion was directly addressed to the European Commissioner for Consumer Health, Tonio Borg. From the outset, this way of challenging public authorities by the scientific community announces the nuance of the discursive framing, which is key to the second period of media coverage analyzed: public authorities are held responsible for implementing regulations, following the scientific literature and considering the difficulties of building evidence involving the long-term consequences of endocrine disruptor use. At a discursive level, using quotations from scientists, the media coverage reflects emerging hypothetical or worrying discourses:

> The signatories [...] say they are "concerned" to see "the prevalence of diseases linked to the hormonal system reaching unprecedented heights [...] in the European Union and worldwide". Among them, the authors cite several cancers (breast, prostate, testis, endometrium, ovary, thyroid), fertility disorders, neuro-behavioral diseases (attention disorders, hyperactivity, etc.), obesity and type 2 diabetes (Foucart 2013).

The matter related to the links between thyroid disease and endocrine-disrupting pesticides remains on the long list of consequences engendered by the use of these substances: several types of cancer. However, the list has now been extended to include other health problems: fertility problems, neurobehavioral disorders, obesity and diabetes. Furthermore, the journalist points out an increase in the incidence of these diseases in humans over the past 30 years or so, while using authoritative arguments to make it clear that "there is growing evidence that environmental factors, including exposure to chemical substances, are involved in these phenomena" (Foucart 2013). A first shift takes place at the discursive level, as concerns are accompanied by the production of evidence. The limits of the existing regulatory tools for assessing the so-called low-dose effects are also pointed out by the journalist, resorting again to arguments of authority by quoting scientists, "some endocrine disruptors have toxicological properties that make it impossible to define thresholds below which exposure can be defined as risk-free" (Foucart 2013).

In line with the scientists' difficulty in producing evidence of the consequences of using these substances, the journalists use quotes from scientists, which function as arguments of authority, and highlights a clear opposition between two types of actors (scientific community and public authorities). Furthermore, they denunciate the impact of the industrial lobby. Quotes from the declaration's signatories provide information on the context in which it was produced. For example, the group chose to limit its signatories to "specialists actively publishing work on the subject", presenting itself as having reached a consensus. The signatories also denounce the public authorities' regulatory failings, which do not keep up the pace with the results of work financed by these same institutions. As they explain, when a new product is launched on the market, manufacturers are not required to carry out tests designed to assess the hormonal activity of the product in question. According to the scientists, this leads to considerable loopholes:

> "The declaration thus represents a consensus of scientists who are at the forefront of knowledge production on the subject. While many of us have received European funding for our work, the knowledge we have accumulated remains ignored by European regulations," says the researcher (Foucart 2013).

In 2014, with the publication of the biologist Barbara Demeneix's work, the discursive register of "concern" moved up a notch to qualify the problem as a "danger" in the journalistic discourse. Demeneix explains the rapid increase in the frequency of neurobehavioral disorders, mainly as a result of the general population's exposure to certain diffuse chemical pollutants, particularly pregnant women and young children. Here, the thyroid takes center stage, as we are specifically talking about substances and "molecules likely to alter the behavior or cognitive capacities of children exposed in utero or in the early stages of life". The journalistic discourse here not only relies on the use of authoritative arguments, citing the scientific community or figures produced by health authorities, but also reinforces these forms of "proof" with quotations from the scientists' peers:

> The problem is that there are so many substances that can disrupt these processes. "Chemists manipulate phenols to which they add halogens such as bromine, chlorine or fluorine," explains Barbara Demeneix. "But thyroid hormones are composed of iodine, which is also a halogen. The result is that we have put into circulation myriads of synthetic substances that closely resemble thyroid hormones" (Foucart 2014).

The more scientific knowledge is acquired, the more alarms are raised and the problem of endocrine disruptors becomes more widespread; from the environment to the food chain, highlighting the multiplicity of consequences: type 2 diabetes, obesity, hormone-dependent cancers (breast, prostate, thyroid) and neurobehavioral disorders (attention deficit disorder, hyperactivity, etc.). By 2015, previous warnings from toxicologists, epidemiologists and biologists were reinforced by reproductive health experts, supported by NGOs (WECF – Women in Europe for a Common Future, and HEAL – Health and Environment Alliance). The International Federation of Gynecology and Obstetrics and the Endocrine Society joined the ranks of those denouncing these effects and accumulating scientific work. All in all, the community of scientific researchers is now joined by the medical community and healthcare professionals in direct contact with patients, at the forefront of what the daily newspaper describes as a "silent health crisis". As a result, the media coverage reflects a change in the discursive framing of journalistic articles, a change that goes hand in hand with the increase of scientific evidence and studies: a discursive register that highlights the transformation of previous "concerns" into "worrying findings", or even "definitive" evidence and a "silent health crisis", demanding a solution from the public authorities in view of the need to review regulations:

> "The evidence for the health damage of endocrine disruptors is more definitive than ever," believes Andrea Gore, Professor of Pharmacology at the University of Texas at Austin, who chaired the group of scientists responsible for drafting the Endocrine Society's

> statement. "Hundreds of studies point in the same direction, from long-term epidemiological studies in humans, to studies in animals and cells, to groups of people exposed to specific products in their jobs" (Foucart and Santi 2015).

However, the link between pesticides that can function as endocrine disruptors, leading to thyroid dysfunction, is not a high-profile issue with a specific name which could help simplify the publicization of the problem as well as its understanding by the newspaper readership. More likely to be publicized as an offshoot of the effects of endocrine disruptors, the problem remains complex, even in the work of the scientific community. It is an issue in a long list of consequences for human health, along with other public health problems (diabetes, obesity, cancers, fertility and reproduction, neurobehavioral disorders, etc.).

6.4.2. *...to denouncing conflicts of interest within European public authorities*

Gradually, the media began to take a stand on the issue, with the publication of editorials that hinted at the daily newspaper's choice to side with the scientific and the medical community in the face of European public powers. A 2015 article describes the regulatory failings of endocrine disruptors as a "major public health risk" and reveals that "the European Commission, which had pledged to give these substances a regulatory definition by December 2013 at the latest, buckled under the weight of lobbying and postponed the implementation of this measure indefinitely" (Le Monde 2015). Another article from 2016 highlights the European Commission's lack of action under the influence of the industrial lobby, going so far as to accuse it of inaction: "given formal notice to react, the European Commission has, on the contrary, gone out of its way to evade the problem, obfuscated expert opinions and postponed any serious decision" (Le Monde 2016). A series of events calling the European Commission's position into question are recalled in evidence in the same article:

> In November 2014, supported by the vast majority of member states and the European Parliament, Sweden brought an action against the European Commission for failure to act before the Court of Justice of the European Union. In December 2015, the Court ruled that the Commission had "infringed the Union law". As recently as January, the President of the European Parliament, Martin Schulz, denounced the Commission's "unacceptable" delay. But to no avail (Le Monde 2016).

The discursive framing, according to which the solution called for is regulation of endocrine disruptors, remains similar. What changes is the pattern of actors involved. The scientific and medical community, joined by associations and NGOs, is now reinforced by the media. This choice of the daily newspaper is gradually becoming clearer and can also be seen in the titles of certain articles: "Europe too lax in the face of the dangers of hundreds of hormone disruptors", May 27, 2013; "Endocrine disruptors: Brussels at fault", May 23, 2016; "Regulation of chemical substances – A denial of scientific consensuses", November 30, 2016, "Endocrine disruptors: France capitulates. A considerable burden for societies and economies", December 6, 2017. These articles were written by journalists specializing in environmental issues, Stéphane Foucart, and *Le Monde* contributor, Stéphane Horel. With this assumed position, a column by Stéphane Foucart goes so far as to use the collective "we", while leaving room for a new discursive development, as the situation is described here as an emergency:

> Brussels has not understood that it is no longer a question of taking precautionary measures, but emergency measures. We can no longer only see this in the rising incidence of "classic" hormonal diseases (hormone-dependent cancers, diabetes, infertility, etc.): our brains and those of future generations, the sine qua non of our collective intelligence, are on the front line (Foucart 2016).

Stéphane Horel's article, "A denial of the scientific consensus" from November 30, 2016, announces the nuance right from the subtitle: "The European Commission has chosen to rely on industry-funded studies". The first element refers to a controversy concerning the scientific data; the results of the EFSA's 2013 opinion, which the European Commission follows, are opposed to the work of the academic society, Endocrine Society, the report of the WHO and the UNEP. The second element relates to conflicts of interest. As the journalist explains,

> In particular, the Commission bases its negative assessments on "critical comments", published in 2014, challenging the methods and conclusions of the WHO/UNEP report. Among its ten authors, seven work for Exponent and Gradient, consulting firms specializing in scientific issues known as "product advocacy companies" (Horel 2016).

Ulrich Beck's observations on the non-tangible and invisible nature of risks are echoed in this controversy. The questioning of scientific legitimacy and scientific expertise are among the arguments used by the opposing camps. Scientific studies are multiplying, and with them, the various actions to challenge European public authorities, such as the letter from Christopher Portier, a toxicologist, biostatistician and former director of several US federal research institutions, addressed to the

President of the European Commission, Jean-Claude Juncker. In this case too, it was a question of scientific studies not being considered by the European Commission. The two journalists reporting on this action, Stéphane Foucart and Stéphane Horel, once again highlight the existence of conflicts of interest within the European authorities:

> The scientist's letter coincides with the gradual publication of the "Monsanto Papers" across the Atlantic, a collection of internal documents from the Missouri-based company. These shed a sometimes-harsh light on the way in which Monsanto has long influenced the glyphosate expertise agencies – those forwarded by the industry to the European authorities. He has uncovered information that had previously gone unnoticed (Le Monde 2017).

Media coverage of the links between endocrine-disrupting pesticides and thyroid diseases continues in the shape of the controversy surrounding the regulation of endocrine disruptors. Thyroid cancer cases are a reminder of the long list of consequences and impacts linked to the use of numerous substances. Amid controversy over the state of scientific knowledge on the subject, the economic damage to health caused by the use of these substances is also beginning to be studied, with estimates of 157 billion euros per year in the European Union. Other studies are investigating the potential impact on brain development, with a particular focus on the future generations and the evolution of IQ. These are revealing new ramifications of the problem. In his investigative work on the subject, the journalist Stéphane Foucart reports on the plurality of these ramifications (cognitive abilities, neurobehavioral disorders) in relation to the impacts of disruptors on the hormones produced by the thyroid gland. Authoritative arguments using quotations, paraphrases and rephrasings, including interviews with scientists such as Barbara Demeneix, are recurrent in support of these statements. Questions related to the exposure of pregnant women and fetuses, or even children, are the subject of several alarming articles. It is difficult to understand whether the problem is environmental, health-related, dietary, or all three. Endocrine disruptors are such a complex issue; it is hard to say. Therefore, it is becoming even more difficult for these links with thyroid dysfunctions to gain visibility in the myriads of issues which are emerging or becoming associated with health problems (diabetes, obesity).

Media coverage continues with the publication of a proposal signed by several scientists in response to statements made by the former Minister of Agriculture, Didier Guillaume, who claims that the obligation to prove that pesticide use has an impact, falls to scientists. The importance of this incident lies, among other things, in the scientists' statements, which rectify these remarks by emphasizing, on the one hand, the legal obligations of industrialists and, on the other hand, that with regard to the "toxic effects of pesticides, scientists have been accumulating evidence for many years, to such an extent that it is no longer necessary to invoke the precautionary principle, but that of prevention" (Le Monde 2018).

Criticized on several occasions, the European Commission's position to the regulation of endocrine disruptors will lead to a certain form of competition with regard to the ownership and definition of the problem, within the European public authorities themselves. Following the European Commission's presentation in November 2018 of its strategy on the regulatory framework for endocrine disruptors, aimed at reducing the population's exposure to substances that are capable of interfering with the hormonal system, the European Parliament commissioned a report on the issue and mandated representatives of the scientific community: Barbara Demeneix (CNRS, French National Museum of Natural History) and Rémy Slama (INSERM, University of Grenoble). Journalist Stéphane Foucart points out that, according to the report by these two scientists, "as it stands, current regulations do not have the means to meet the objectives set by the European executive" (Foucart 2019).

Through the regular use of quotations, the journalistic article reflects an effort to centralize the numerous arguments put forward by the scientific community:

– The discrepancy between regulations and the state of knowledge, due to the failure to consider the cumulative effects of these substances on exposed populations, such as the cocktail effect: "in the majority of regulatory texts, each molecule is considered one by one, independently of the others".

– Inconsistencies between different regulations, with some incorporating the notion of endocrine disruptor, while others do not.

– The need to include a definition of endocrine disruptors for all sectors that are potentially involved and to rapidly develop regulatory tests capable of identifying them, adopting, for example, for carcinogens, three levels of proof: suspected, presumed, proven. "Current scientific knowledge, accumulated over more than 30 years, is sufficient to justify these recommendations".

The last major subject to receive media coverage in the period under review was journalist Stéphane Horel's investigation into chlorpyrifos, a family of pesticides with impacts on the central nervous system and intelligence quotient. Used as an insecticide, it is, according to the data provided by the journalist, an endocrine disrupter that interacts with the thyroid axis and can lead to delayed mental development, reduced working memory and attention deficit disorders with (or without) hyperactivity. In the context in which the European Commission was preparing to propose the withdrawal of this substance from the market, the journalist's investigation highlights that the authorities took almost 20 years before assessing the data from the manufacturer, Dow. In fact, as early as 2014, a "chlorpyrifos task force", set up by Dow and other manufacturers, had submitted a file requesting renewal of the insecticide to the EFSA. Responsible for the process, the agency delegated the examination of the file to a "rapporteur member state" – Spain. As a counterpoint, the NGO *Générations Futures* has also taken the matter into its own hands. Based on the work of this NGO, the journalist explains that only 131 existing scientific studies were taken into account by the task force. Supported by evidence, the journalist explains the NGO's approach, which, "by searching PubMed, one of the main databases of scientific publications [...] found 1,023 studies dealing with the toxicity of chlorpyrifos, published between 2006 and 2017" (Horel 2019). Against this statement of scientific ignorance and the creation of doubt[3], the counter-arguments put forward by the rapporteur member state are also presented, according to which "the disparate results (final number of relevant and reliable references) [...] seem to show that the research strategies applied were not appropriate" (Horel 2019). In a back-and-forth presentation of arguments and counter-arguments, the journalist goes on to highlight the conflicts of interest between public authorities and industry. As she explains:

> But the chlorpyrifos file consists, above all, of a series of studies, almost all of which were carried out or financed by Dow and others. Following the glyphosate saga, the public was stunned to discover that EFSA was placing its trust in industrialists who have no interest in presenting their product in a disadvantageous light. Yet, although there are suspicions, no one has ever been able to gauge these manufacturers' studies and their possible biases: they are confidential, protected by commercial secrecy (Horel 2019).

6.5. Conclusion

Over the last 10 years or so, *Le Monde* has published articles on pesticides that can disrupt thyroid function. While this media coverage is closely linked to developments in the publication of knowledge by the scientific community, these are not articles solely dealing with thyroid-related issues. Indeed, in the context of accumulating scientific knowledge, thyroid, and the various other dysfunctions associated with it, join the long list of health problems, in which endocrine disruptors play a part. The analysis shows that the media coverage can be divided into two periods: one before 2013, when the few articles published in the press mainly reported on the links between pesticides' use and various types of cancer, including thyroid cancer and another after 2013, when scientific knowledge on endocrine disruptors became more accurate and accumulated, revealing numerous ramifications, ranging from the environment to food and health: atmospheric pollution, neurobehavioral disorders, reproduction and fertility, diabetes, obesity and

3 See also the works of Foucart et al. (2020).

more. An analysis of media coverage of the endocrine disruptors highlights the difficulty of naming the problem related to the links between pesticides and thyroid dysfunctions. It is not easy to publicize a problem without being able to name it. As the journalist Stéphane Foucart himself points out in connection with the film Dark Waters and the publicization of the consequences of chemical use: "one of the reasons for this is that certain health or environmental scandals are, in the literal sense of the word, indescribable. There are no intelligible words or concrete situations to tell the story" (Foucart 2020).

Another element highlighted by the analysis relates to the problem's publicization pattern, as well as to the discursive framing used in the media coverage process. Indeed, the scientific and medical community, joined by associations and NGOs, is also supported by the daily newspaper, with the editorials clearly showing its positioning on the subject in favor of the scientific community. Competitive struggles over the ownership of the problem's definition by European public authorities can also be observed. The discursive framing that emerges reveals a plurality of health problems linked to the use of so-called endocrine disruptors. The European Union's public institutions are held responsible for providing a solution. This includes updating regulations that are supported, at a discursive level of articles, by a register which evolves and shows a progressive transformation. Gradually, "concerns" become "worrying facts", before giving way to formulations such as "definitive" evidence, or even a "silent health crisis" and an "emergency", to name the problem. Several articles report on conflicts of interest within the public authorities, related to the lobbying activities of industrialists, ranging from denunciations to accusations of inaction of public authorities in implementing regulations.

The relatively recent problem of pesticides disrupting the thyroid gland has received little media coverage. The complexity of health, environmental and dietary problems, to which the issue refers, makes it difficult to name the problem. Nonetheless, media coverage does demonstrate a genuine investigative effort to publicize the complexity of the problems associated with endocrine-disrupting pesticides, among other things, through regular recourse to scientific sources. In short, at this stage, it is a problem that is mainly being addressed by the scientific community, calling on European public authorities to strengthen the regulation framework. However, as Emmanuel Henry points out, the tendency "to analyze the role of expertise as a pivot between scientific knowledge and public decisions" (Henry 2021, p. 78) does not quite mirror the real process. Our analysis has shown that this is also not the case for thyroid endocrine disruptors. Therefore, future work aims to extend the results of this initial work, relating it to work on the "creation of ignorance" (Oreskes and Conway 2014).

6.6. References

Ackerman, G., Grandazzi, G., Lemarchand, F. (2006). *Les silences de Tchernobyl*. Autrement, Paris.

Alliance pour les chiffres de la presse et des médias (ACPM) (2022). Classement diffusion presse quotidienne nationale [Online]. Available at: http://www.acpm.fr/Les-chiffres/Diffusion-Presse/Presse-Payante/Presse-Quotidienne-Nationale [Accessed February 21, 2022].

ANSES (2014). Étude de l'alimentation totale (EAT 2) : l'Anses met à disposition les données de son analyse interrégionale de l'exposition aux substances [Online]. Available at: https://www.anses.fr/fr/content/%C3%A9tude-de-l%E2%80%99alimentation-totale-eat-2-l%E2%80%99anses-met-%C3%A0-disposition-les-donn%C3%A9es-de-son-analyse [Accessed 28 August 2022].

Arquembourg, J. (2016a). L'antibiorésistance, un problème en quête de publics. *Questions de communication*, 29, 7–134.

Arquembourg, J. (2016b). Analyse d'un processus inachevé de constitution d'un problème public. *Questions de communication*, 29, 29–48.

Badau, E. (2019). De la mise à l'épreuve de l'alimentation par l'antibiorésistance au développement des concepts sans antibiotique et One Health : publicisation et communication en France et aux États-Unis. PhD Thesis, Université Sorbonne Nouvelle – Paris 3, Paris.

Badau, E., Fortané, N., Arquembourg, J. (2022). Les appropriations de l'antibiorésistance en France : la carrière d'un problème public au sein de la presse vétérinaire. In *Croisades privés et problèmes publics. L'héritage sociologique de Joseph Gusfield*, Bernardin, S. (ed.). PUR, Rennes, 217–232.

Beck, U. (2008). *La société du risque. Sur la voie d'une autre modernité*. Flammarion. Paris.

Boudia, S. and Jas, N. (2019). *Gouverner un monde toxique*. Quae, Versailles.

Cefaï, D. (1996). La construction des problèmes publics. Définitions de situations dans des arènes publiques. *Réseaux*, 14(75), 43–66.

Cefaï, D. (2016). Publics, problèmes publics, arènes publiques… Que nous apprend le pragmatisme ? *Questions de communication*, 30, 25–64.

Cessou, S. (2005). Tchernobyl : le déni français. *Alternatives Internationales*, 26(8), 40.

Chateauraynaud, F. (2014). Trajectoires argumentatives et constellations discursives. Exploration socio-informatique des futurs vus depuis le nanomonde. *Réseaux*, 188(6), 121–158.

EFSA (2013). Scientific Opinion on the identification of pesticides to be included in cumulative assessment groups on the basis of their toxicological profile. *EFSA Journal*, 11(7) [Online]. Available at: https://www.efsa.europa.eu/fr/efsajournal/pub/3293 [Accessed 28 August 2022].

Entman, R. (1993). Framing: Toward clarification of a fractured paradigm. *Journal of Communication*, 43(4), 51–58.

Erbs, V. and Joubert, A. (2017). Les perturbateurs endocriniens et la glande thyroïde. *Environnement, risques et santé*, 16(6), 583–590.

Fischer, G.-N. and Tarquinio, C. (2014). La maladie : aspects psychosociaux. In *Les concepts fondamentaux de la psychologie de la santé*, Fischer, G.-N. and Tarquinio, C. (eds). Dunod, Paris, 135–161.

Foucart, S. (2013). L'Europe trop laxiste face aux dangers de centaines de perturbateurs hormonaux. *Le Monde*.

Foucart, S. (2014). Le cerveau en danger. *Le Monde*.

Foucart, S. (2016). Le cerveau assiégé. *Le Monde*.

Foucart, S. (2019). L'UE tarde à réguler les perturbateurs endocriniens. *Le Monde*.

Foucart, S. (2020). Perfluorés en eaux troubles. *Le Monde*.

Foucart, S. and Horel, S. (2017). Glyphosate et cancer : des études-clés sous-estimées. *Le Monde*.

Foucart, S. and Santi, P. (2015). Environnement : les enfants naissent pré-pollués. *Le Monde*.

Foucart, S., Horel, S., Laurens, S. (2020). *Les gardiens de la raison. Enquête sur la désinformation scientifique*. La Découverte, Paris.

Générations Futures (2021a). Pesticides Perturbateurs endocriniens : Il faut agir ! [Online]. Available at: https://www.generations-futures.fr/wp-content/uploads/2022/03/version-finale-rapport-pe-thyroide-vol2.pdf [Accessed 28 August 2022].

Générations Futures (2021b). Pesticides Perturbateurs endocriniens : Il est temps d'agir ! [Online]. Available at: https://www.generations-futures.fr/wp-content/uploads/2021/04/rapport-thyroide-v9.pdf [Accessed 28 August 2022].

Générations Futures (2022). Pesticides Perturbateurs endocriniens : Il faut agir ! [Online]. Available at: https://www.generations-futures.fr/actualites/perturbateur-thyroidien/ [Accessed 28 August 2022].

Goldner, W.S., Sandler, D.P., Yu, F., Hoppin, J.A., Kamel, F., LeVan, T.D. (2010). Pesticide use and thyroid disease among women in the agricultural health study. *American Journal of Epidemiology*, 171(4), 455–464.

Gusfield, J. (1981). *The Culture of Public Problems. Drinking-Driving and the Symbolic Order*. The University of Chicago Press, Chicago.

Gusfield, J. (1996). *Contested Meanings. The Construction of Alcohol Problems*. The University of Wisconsin Press, Madison.

Henry, E. (2021). *La fabrique de non-problèmes ou comment éviter que la politique s'en mêle*. Presses de Sciences Po, Paris.

Horel, S. (2016). Un déni du consensus scientifique. *Le Monde*.

Horel, S. (2019). Chlorpyrifos, une toxicité passée sous silence. *Le Monde.*

Huet, S. (2020). Les sciences du vivant dans les médias. Quelques mécanismes à l'origine de mal-information en sciences de la vie. *Raison présente*, 2–3(214–215), 131–137.

Le Monde (2015). Le poison invisible de la pollution chimique. *Le Monde.*

Le Monde (2016). Perturbateurs endocriniens : Bruxelles en faute. *Le Monde.*

Le Monde (2017). Perturbateurs endocriniens : la France capitule. Un fardeau considérable pour les sociétés et les économies, *Le Monde.*

Le Monde (2018). Collectif : notre proposition, monsieur le ministre, pour évaluer la toxicité des pesticides. *Le Monde.*

Lewandowski, C. (2021). Les accidents nucléaires et leurs enseignements. In *Le nucléaire*, Lewandowski, C. (ed.). PUF, Paris, 34–42.

Maingueneau, D. (1987). *Nouvelles tendances en analyse du discours.* Hachette, Paris.

Moirand, S. (2007). *Les discours de la presse quotidienne. Observer, analyser, comprendre.* PUF, Paris.

Moreau, Y. (2019). La terre et les rêveries de la volonté, à Fukushima. *Communications*, 2(105), 235–246.

Niel, J.-C. and Couturier, J. (2020). Que s'est-il passé à Three Mile Island, Tchernobyl et Fukushima Daiichi ? Et où en est-on aujourd'hui ? *Responsabilité et environnement, annales des mines*, 1(97), 25–30.

Oreskes, N. and Conway, E.M. (2014). *Les marchands de doute. Ou comment une poignée de scientifiques ont masqué la vérité sur des enjeux de société tels que le tabagisme et le réchauffement climatique.* Le Pommier, Paris.

Orsini, S. (2004). Le cancer de la thyroïde, un cancer à part. In *Le cancer : approche psychodynamique chez l'adulte*, Ben Soussan, P. (ed.). Érès, Toulouse, 173–178.

Pailliart, I. (2005). *La publicisation de la science. Exposer, communiquer, débattre, publier, vulgariser.* PUG, Grenoble.

Pena-Vega, A. (2002). Les incertitudes de l'incident de Tchernobyl. L'émergence du sens dans les territoires contaminés en Belarus. *Sociétés*, 3(77), 37–54.

Pigement, C. (2019). *Levothyrox : une scandaleuse négligence.* Archipel, Paris.

Pugeat, M. (2017). Fonction thyroïdienne et perturbateurs endocriniens. Fédération d'Endocrinologie du Pôle Est Hospices Civils de Lyon et INSERM U1060 Institut CaRMeN.

Vitaux, J. and Spielrein, M. (2015). Alimentation et cancers. In *Au risque de manger*, Vitaux, J. and Spielrein, M. (eds). PUF, Paris, 263–265.

Voirol, O. (2005). Les luttes pour la visibilité. Esquisse d'une problématique. *Réseaux*, 1–2(129–130), 89–121.

7

Discursive Strategies of a Sociotechnical Network: The Case of Natural Plant Defense Stimulators

7.1. Introduction

For decades, chemical and biological control have structured the field of plant protection in France, with the latter's economic and political significance being linked to its balance of trade and food sovereignty. In this context, the development of natural plant defense stimulators (*stimulateurs des défenses naturelles des plantes* (SDN)) is something of an anomaly. Also known as "plant vaccines", SDNs are unique in that they help plants defend themselves against fungi and bacteria, rather than attacking them directly. They thus circumvent pest control, providing an environmentally friendly solution. The analytical framework of science and technology studies has, in the past, enabled us to follow the sociotechnical network of SDNs across the laboratory, the market, regulatory bodies and farmers (Blanchard 2016, 2018a).

To complete this work, in this chapter, we suggest using discourse analysis to identify the discursive strategies of this sociotechnical network. Considering discourse as an act of communication involving linguistic and textual structures (Maingueneau 2014), we will use both quantitative approaches from content analysis (Berelson 1952) and qualitative approaches used in linguistics.

Our main hypothesis is that, between 1997 and 2007, the communication of SDNs fulfilled a dual strategy of promises and demarcation, through five singular areas of communication: scientific literature, technical and marketing documentation, the trade press, the general public press and the popular science and

Chapter written by Antoine BLANCHARD.

technology press. In these different corpora, we seek to show how the discursive strategy of SDNs contrasts with the terminology and discursive treatment of other categories of plant protection products, including closely related biopesticides.

For scientific literature, we collected academic articles on SDNs published in English between 1994 and 2008, from various bibliographic databases. For technical and marketing documentation, we focused on the *Index Acta phytosanitaire* published by the *Association de coordination technique Agricole* (Agricultural technical coordination association (ACTA)). For the trade press, we perused the tables of content of the *Phytoma – La Défense des végétaux* journal and searched their web database to identify 12 articles devoted to SDNs over the 1997–2007 period. For the daily and weekly press, we searched the Europresse database for 43 articles in French, published between 1997 and 2007. For the popular press, we accumulated six articles on SDNs published between 1993 and 2007.

Section 7.2 looks back at SDNs, initially from a technical point of view, then from the perspective of the sociology of translation, before describing the method used for discourse analysis. Section 7.3 looks at the term *SDN*, which has become an established part of our vocabulary. Section 7.4 looks at the various areas of communication mentioned above. Before concluding, a final section (section 7.5) compares this discursive treatment with that of biopesticides.

7.2. The role of SDNs in the field of plant protection

Noting "the unintended effects of synthetic organic pesticides [and the urgent need] to propose 'ecologically sound' alternative solutions" (Philogène et al. 2005, pp. 6–7), the public policy to reduce pesticide use in France has included a focus on promoting "natural" alternatives to synthetic pesticides (Pellissier 2021, pp. 303–307). One particular family of pesticides has benefited from this strategy: natural plant defense stimulators (SDNs). Like vaccines, SDNs simulate an attack or activate innate defense mechanisms, which can then react faster and more effectively to the next real attack.

In 2002, the French *Larousse agricole* defined SDNs as:

> Substances which, when applied to plants, trigger defense mechanisms that can later be effective against parasitic attacks. Being of various natures (polysaccharides, enzymes), SDNs act as elicitors and are capable of reinforcing plant resistance to attackers, particularly fungi. They could be of particular interest in organic farming, but also in industrial agriculture, as a back-up to conventional treatments.

This definition, contemporary with the corpus under study here, shows how SDNs are described through their elicitor role (the ability to trigger plant defense reactions), regardless of their biological or chemical nature: living microorganisms, proteins, simple, complex or inorganic chemical substances, etc.

In Alan Wood's *Compendium of Pesticide Common Names*, which is an authoritative resource for professionals and researchers alike, SDNs form a separate category, that of "plant activators". SDNs are sometimes simply overlooked in reviews, such as Marcos Kogan's (1998) review on integrated protection in the *Annual Review of Entomology*. They may also suffer from a certain similarity to other alternative control methods such as biopesticides (which will be discussed in detail later) or semiochemical control, which "covers the use of any chemical compound emitted by plants, animals and other organisms, as well as synthetic analogues, which modify the physiology or behavior of individuals of the same or different species" (Philogène et al. 2005, pp. 9–10). These issues regarding terminology are the focus of this chapter.

7.2.1. *Discursive strategies at the service of a sociotechnical network*

Historical work has enabled us to document how SDNs were formed in the laboratory, in line with plant pathology research on plant defense reactions, and how they collided with the plant protection industry, which was largely focused on chemical research and not on biological techniques (Blanchard 2018a). Epistemological analysis has led us to show how SDNs have forced preexisting epistemic communities to reposition themselves, and how they have split communities that were previously mixed: molecular biologists and agronomists, academic engineers and researchers, small and medium-sized enterprises (SMEs) and multinational agrochemical companies (Blanchard 2016). In both cases, using actor-network theory (Callon 1986; Latour 1997), we followed translation chains, which are described as a subtle interplay of equivalences "between problems formulated by several actors in different repertoires", in order to link together "the various human and non-human actors involved in the formulation of these problems and their resolution" (Callon and Law 1989, p. 81).

To become established, SDN translation chains have to come to terms with the sociotechnical systems of chemical and biological control, which have been at odds with one another for decades in the world of plant protection. According to the definitions cited above, SDNs are at a minimum recognized by their effect on the plant. This definition distinguishes them from biological and chemical control, both of which are concerned with the pest rather than the plant. However, biological and chemical controls are differentiated by the nature of the agent used to obtain this effect. As a result, SDNs have a common factor with each of the other two plant protection paradigms: the nature of the agent. Some complex biologically derived SDNs, such as polyglucans, cannot be synthesized chemically, and could therefore fit into the biological control paradigm: in its broadest definition, this goes beyond using living auxiliary organisms such as ladybugs (known as "classical biological control") to instead "using any biological organisms and products" (Philogène et al. 2005, p. 9). Other SDNs, such as acibenzolar-S-methyl, have long been domesticated by synthesis processes used in laboratories and factories that are closer to chemical control (Blanchard 2016). Instead of fitting into one of these two systems, the natural defense stimulation competes with them in a third way.

To translate is also to derive, to betray and to be ambiguous: "translation is always, by definition, a misunderstanding, since we find common interests that are, in the long run, bound to diverge" (Callon and Law 1989, p. 108). By trying too hard to appeal to an ever-increasing variety of actors, SDNs could weaken and disappear. Another danger facing SDNs is that of being caught up in a larger movement, that of integrated pest management. Pierre Jourdheuil et al. (1991) note, for example, that the "climate of controversy and misunderstanding" between chemical and biological control has "faded considerably" since the advent of integrated pest management. There are therefore several outcomes for the SDN sociotechnical network: to exist in its own right, or to merge with another cause.

We therefore expect discourses on SDNs to serve two functions. On the one hand, they are part of an economy of promise as described by economic sociology, in other words, a way for the SDN sociotechnical network to organize market expectations and use them to shape the development and future of its technology. This promise makes it possible to set medium- and long-term objectives, in order to attract the attention of politicians and lawmakers, and to obtain the means to work (funding, etc.). It has a powerful appeal, since it describes "a completely different world", in the words of a Syngenta engineer we interviewed, a world where all plant protection problems would be solved. On the other hand, discourses on SDNs mark a boundary between this sociotechnical network and those of chemical control, biological control and even integrated protection. This distinction is still the subject of constant study (referred to as "boundary work"), and the result of rhetorical and institutional investments.

The aim of this chapter is to show how these two objectives of promise and boundary combine to give a unique tone to SDN communication, through five distinct areas of communication.

7.2.2. *Discourse analysis method and corpus*

Based on a multidisciplinary approach, this chapter uses the study of vocabulary and discourse to support hypotheses from the social studies of science and technology, which combine historical and sociological approaches to understand how science, technology and social issues intermingle and relate to one another. The corpora studied range from 1997, when the term *SDN* was introduced at an international congress on plant diseases (Blanchard 2018a), to 2007, when the Grenelle de l'environnement launched the Écophyto 2018 program, which aimed to halve the amount of pesticide treatments over the next 10 years, withdrawing the most toxic substances from the French market. This decision came from two major milestones:

– In 2006, the French agricultural policy law extinguished industry hopes of simplifying the marketing authorization procedure for products that "intended to exert an action on vital plant processes [such as defense reactions], insofar as they are not nutrients [such as fertilizers]". This law led to the so-called "nettle manure" case (Blanchard 2018a).

– Also in 2006, the inter-ministerial pesticide risk reduction plan (PIRRP) made the reduction of pesticide use and the associated health risks a public policy objective (Pellissier 2021, pp. 285–286).

The year 2007 was therefore a key year, ushering in an era in which SDNs were subjected to a harsh economic reality (with no simplified approval process and no derogation regime), even though pesticide use had to be reduced. Prior to this date, between 1997 and 2007, the SDN sociotechnical network had spent a decade considering plant vaccines as a credible alternative to pesticides.

Each corpus studied corresponds to a single area of communication, namely, in order: scientific literature, technical and marketing documentation, the trade press, the general public press and the popular scientific and technology press. Outside of these corpora, we occasionally refer to interviews conducted during our science and technology study, as described in a previous article (Blanchard 2018a).

7.2.3. *A hegemonic term*

"To name a thing is to affirm its existence, and [...] to impose it on others" (Mortureux 1984). Studying this act of language allows us to understand how things play a role in the public arena, as a social referent signifying something for everyone.

In this case, the phrase "natural defense stimulator" and its acronym SDN bring together all of the actors surrounding it, be it SMEs investing in research and development (R&D), trade associations calling for a more flexible regulatory framework, farmers turning to alternative solutions to pesticides, researchers seeking funding for their projects, etc.

Despite their differences and sometimes their clashes, they all claim to be SDNs, which has become an obligatory part of their vocabulary, like the "sustainable development" formula studied by Alice Krieg-Planque (2010) (only the "elicitor" has managed to coexist, to a lesser extent). By using this name, each actor recognizes that they are not isolated, but part of a network that is capable of ensuring the sustainability of SDNs.

Furthermore, the phrase "natural defense stimulator" has the advantage of being easy to understand, since it is made up of everyday terms, despite the fact that they take on a specialized meaning, as is often the case in scientific discourse.

On the contrary, there are six competing expressions in English: "SAR inducing compound", "SAR inducer", "plant activator", "systemic inducer", "resistance promoter" and "natural defense stimulator"; and four in German: "resistenz-induzierende Natursubstanz", "Pflänzenstärkungsmittel", "Elicitor" and "Resistenzinduktor" (Blanchard 2018a). In both languages, mixed terminology does not help us to form a common understanding.

From a constructivist linguistic perspective, the existence of the SDN category is thus reinforced by this clear and widely adopted naming, which also has the advantage of clearly delineating this discourse study.

7.3. Specificity of SDNs in areas of communication

7.3.1. *Study of scientific literature (1994–2008)*

If to name something is to give it the right to exist in the real world, to predicate is to "say something" about that object in the world. Between 1994 and 2008 (the time frame of this corpus), SDNs were still little known, and research publications had to borrow common terminology to be understood by readers: a good predicate then made it possible, in a few words, to characterize them. Following Francesco Attruia's (2020) example of predication in the European Union's institutional discourses on biodiversity, it is informative to study how SDNs are referred to in English scientific literature (see Table 7.1).

What SDNs subsume	
"new class"	Lucas (1999)
"new product category"	Rossignol et al. (1997)
What they do	
"new mode of action"	Lucas (1999)
"new tools"	Klarzynski et al. (2003)
"new technology"	Oostendorp et al. (2001)
How they are forcing us to rethink plant protection	
"new concept"	Kunz et al. (1997) and Fournier (2006)
"new principle"	Kessmann et al. (1994)
"alternative or additional method"	Cole (2008)
"new strategy"	Klarzynski and Fritig (2001)
"new opportunities"	Lyon and Newton (1997)
"new horizons"	Edreva (2004)
"field of research"	Kidd (2002)

Table 7.1. *SDN predication in scientific literature*

A first series of predicates simply recalls how SDNs form a "new class" or "new product category", encompassing a number of substances. A second series of predicates reminds us that behind SDNs lies a phenomenology of "mode of action", "tools" and "technology". Lastly, a third series of predicates establishes the discourse in an axiological manner, by making SDNs a tipping point through the notions of "concept", "principle", "method", "strategy", "opportunities", "horizons" or "field of research".

Almost systematically, the noun phrase presented in the first column of Table 7.1 includes the qualifier term "new", which emphasizes the diverging nature of SDNs, whose consequences are not all laid out, both in 1994 and in 2006. In one of the two cases where this qualifier is absent, it is replaced by the qualifier term "alternative or additional", introducing the notion of complementarity and substitution, to which we will return later.

This last set of predicates leads us to think of SDNs as a new paradigm, in other words, a new way of thinking about pest control like never before. The paradigm concept was first introduced by Thomas Kuhn in 1962 in *The Structure of Scientific Revolutions*, without excessive formalization. It was only in the afterword to the second edition, published in 1970, that he distinguished two different meanings: the first, which he called his "sociological sense", and the second, which "denoted an isolated element of this whole", in other words, "the concrete solutions to riddles which, when used as models or examples, can replace explicit rules as the basis of solutions to the riddles that remain in normal science" (Kuhn 1983). In this second sense, the SDN object serves as a cognitive shortcut for a solution to a phytosanitary problem. For example, a skilled person who visits a field to determine their control strategy or who formulates recommendations for winegrowers, will think of the term "SDN" to encompass "salicylic acid defense pathway", "low environmental impact ", "resistance avoidance", "preventive application", etc. By doing this, they will not be thinking of the terms "chemical control" or "biological control", the other two major competing paradigms. Each of these is also a cognitive shortcut for a wide range of constraints and technical solutions to the various issues (regulatory, agronomic, environmental, societal, economic) that arise in the field of plant protection.

7.3.2. *Study of technical and marketing documentation (1997–2007)*

To be distributed, an SDN must follow current marketing practices, in particular by being broken down into marketing specialties that will appear in the documentation made available to farmers and technical advisors. As this corpus is highly heterogeneous and poorly structured, we have focused on the *Index Acta phytosanitaire*, published annually by the ACTA. Paule Yacoub (2021) reminds us that this association, which was "created in 1956 by professional agricultural organizations, […] is notably responsible for publishing numerous technical aids for advisors, including […] indexes listing the plant protection products that are available on the market", such as the one we analyzed.

What discursive strategy, particularly in terms of onomastics, is adopted in this corpus? One lexical phenomenon stands out: the omnipresence of trademarks (see Table 7.2), no doubt for the same reasons as in industry, where they aim to "designate the product more easily" and "differentiate it from other similar and competing products" (Fèvre-Pernet and Roché 2005). Even when obtained from natural animal or plant extracts, SDNs are viewed in terms of their significance (Fèvre-Pernet and Roché 2005) and marketed under trade names or even trademarks, as is customary in the chemical control and drug industries (Leblanc and Bilodeau 2007).

Trade name	Active substance
Bion® or Actigard®	Acibenzolar-S-methyl
Elexa® or AgroChit®	Chitosan
Iodus 40®	Laminarin
Messenger®	Harpin
Milsana®	*Reynoutria sachalinensis* plant extract
Proradix®	Extract of the bacterium *Pseudomonas fluorescens ssp. proradix*
Sémafort®	Algae extracts, amino acids and fertilizers
Stifénia® or Stimulia®	Fenugreek seed extract
Stimulase®	Purified enzymes from the bacterium *Trichoderma*

Table 7.2. *Some SDN trade names*

Reaching the limits of their boundary work, SDNs are thus forced to adopt current trade names. We would rather see them as natural substances that are easily comprehensible on the market, through their unambiguous origin, but they circulate based on trade agreements and must be available in infinite ranges. Within the multinational company Syngenta, Bion® was associated with the fungicide department, not to an SDN or alternative control strategies department. The company believes that the future of SDNs lies in mixing with traditional fungicides, such as Bion M® used in Asia on vegetable crops, which is a blend between the SDN acibenzolar S methyl and the fungicide mancozeb (Leadbeater and Staub 2007).

The only margin of freedom that SDNs have is on the product label, whose graphic codes show that they are a member of the SDN family. Bion MX®, a fungicide composed of 38.76% mefenoxam fungicide and only 4% acibenzolar-S-methyl, claims a fungicidal effect on its label (in accordance with its marketing authorization), while its stylized leaf logo and slogan “The Plant Activator” serve as a reminder that it is an SDN.

7.3.3. *Study of the trade press (1997–2007)*

In addition to technical and marketing documentation, prescribers (agricultural engineers, technical advisors, etc.) in the crop protection industry read the French magazine *Phytoma – La Défense des végétaux*, which acts as a “link between research and the field” (Bouron et al. 1998, p. 14). *Phytoma* is the result of a 1991 merger between the *Phytoma* and *La Défense des végétaux* magazines. The former was founded in 1945 "by the Comité de Propagande pour la Défense des Cultures, a group of product manufacturers' unions, joined in 1952 by the *Société française de phytiatrie et de phytopharmacie*", and received the patronage of the French Ministry of Agriculture in 1953 (Fourche 2004, p. 385). The second came about in 1947 under the aegis of the *Ligue nationale de lutte contre les ennemis des cultures* (French National Pest Control League), created by top-level scientists and agronomists to "inform users, as candidly as possible, about pest control products and treatment equipment" and to "popularize the best methods for controlling crop pests" (Fourche 2004, p. 306). The product of this merger lays between the authorities, industry, scientists and farmers. In 1998, a survey revealed that its authors were evenly divided between researchers at research organization INRA (now INRAE), plant protection services, technical institutes, industry and a miscellaneous category, while its 25,000 readers were mainly advisors and influential farmers (Bouron et al. 1998).

A manual review of the magazine's summaries and a search of the database, which is accessible on its website, reveal 12 articles devoted to SDNs in *Phytoma*, published regularly over the 1997–2007 period (Blanchard 2016). An analysis of the authors of the articles show that their presence is not due to heavyweight companies of the plant protection industry such as Syngenta or BASF, but rather to research laboratories and the myriad of small companies that occupy "these niches [...] neglected by the major groups, notably because of the importance of (unpatentable) expertise in the organic sector" (Fixari and Hatchuel 1998, p. 349). These SMEs have several characteristics: they are small companies, working in niche markets that are close to farmers. They are sometimes fragile and sometimes disappear or change names. However, they can also be start-ups, i.e. young innovative companies, just like *Science & vie* describes Tribo Technologies[1]. This being said, we have to agree with Stéphane Lemarié et al. (2001, p. 17): there are very few start-up SMEs – in other words, those with intensive research activity – in the agrochemical sector, since they have to deal with the whole development chain and, more often than not, delegate their research to public sector partnerships. Tribo Technologies, for example, would be nothing without its collaboration with the Strasbourg research laboratory, the *Institut de biologie moléculaire des plantes* (French Institute for Plant Molecular Biology). Nonetheless, these SMEs have a different approach to the larger companies, which instead have a "reductionist" (Joly and Lemarié 2002, p. 265) one-problem/one-solution approach, as evidenced by their organization into departments devoted to a single objective (fungicide, herbicide or insecticide), based on routine screening tests (Joly and Lemarié 2002, p. 262). It is undoubtedly because the survival of SMEs directly depends on the

1 Haentjens, E. (2007). On sait enfin vacciner les plantes. *Science & vie*, October, 90–95.

agronomic and commercial success of SDNs, that they are more invested than the major agrochemical multinational companies in this area of communication.

Moreover, this corpus of articles in the *Phytoma* magazine highlights the fact that SDNs have a specific role: according to Pajot et al. (2007), "if results are conclusive, [the use of SDNs] would halve the use of conventional fungicides, thus contributing to the objective of reducing pesticide use set out in the inter-ministerial plan of June 2006". This statement, which opts for cohabitation with chemical control and supports the substitution of a number of treatments, but not of the active ingredients, is not self-evident. The same is true of a press release from the Breton company Goëmar, dated February 24, 2003, which explains that "laminarin is a natural product and, on cereals, it replaces a chemical treatment usually carried out with synthetic active ingredients". An engineer from Arvalis (an institute representing the plant production sector) goes even further, asserting that laminarin can "replace a chemical treatment, or even reduce the application doses of the next one".

Historically, this motto stems from an idea that took off in the early 1990s, when integrated vineyard management no longer just became a question of combining chemical and biological control, or of new, less harmful active substances, but of "reducing the number of sprays and respecting certain auxiliaries" (Fourche 2004, p. 300). Simultaneously, at the end of the 1990s, SDN specialists began to argue that SDNs should be seen as an additional option within the framework of integrated protection, rather than a substitute for fungicides (Lyon and Newton 1999).

The recurrence of this term elicits a community of practice which, according to the inventor of this concept, Etienne Wenger (1999), is made up of a common repertoire that has been produced or integrated over time: routines, words, gestures, symbols, actions or slogans. This common repertoire harmonizes the meaning of knowledge used by the network, and its repetition reinforces its impact in communication. The same term was also relayed by the daily press in the early 2000s, as we will show later. This discursive strategy is therefore an important translation for the SDN network.

7.3.4. *Study of the daily and weekly press (1997–2007)*

A corpus of 43 articles from the French daily and weekly press, published between 1997 and 2007, was compiled from a query on the Europresse database in September 2021, using the following search equation:

TEXT = (stimul* $4 défense+ naturelle+ $3 plante*) | (vaccin* $3 plante+)

The 43 articles are classified manually according to the category of the magazine in which they appear. Figure 7.1 shows that the most articles come from the regional daily press ("Regional" category), ahead of the economic press represented by *La Tribune* and *Les Echos*, and mainstream publications such as *Le Monde*, *Le Point*, *L'Express*, *La Croix* and *Le Figaro*.

The "Professional" category is in light blue for two magazines specializing in the environment, and "Canada" in dark blue for the Quebec press. This unexpected predominance of the regional and economic press is related to the themes of the articles, as we shall see later.

Chronologically speaking, Figure 7.2 shows that the annual number of articles was highest between 2004 and 2007, driven by the regional press, after an initial peak in 2001, which was mostly driven by the economic press.

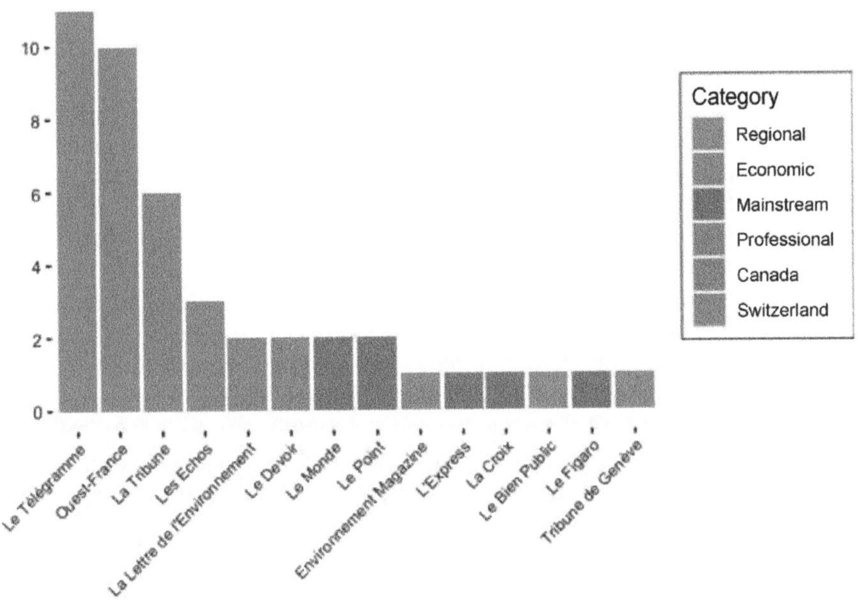

Figure 7.1. *Number of articles on SDNs by news outlet and category. For a color version of this figure, see: www.iste.co.uk/botero/pesticides.zip*

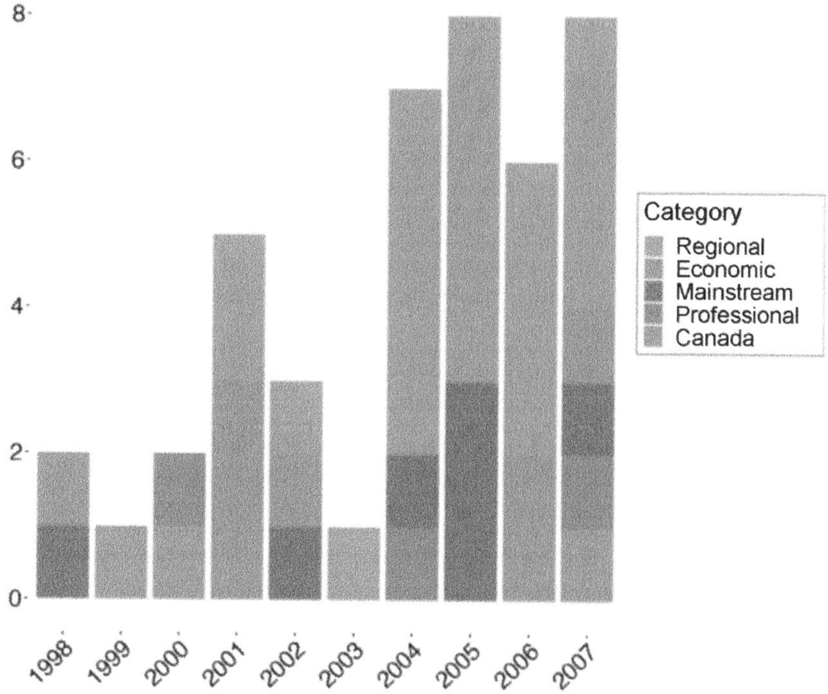

Figure 7.2. *Number of articles on SDNs by year and category. For a color version of this figure, see: www.iste.co.uk/botero/pesticides.zip*

Press articles directly shape the public image of SDNs, much more than the previous two media categories. The theme of each article, and therefore the angle from which the SDNs are treated, plays a key role in shaping their image. A content analysis, in other words, "an objective, systematic and quantitative description of the manifest content of communication" (Berelson 1952), is necessary if we are to understand the system of representations they construct and convey.

Manual coding was used to assign a predominant theme or tone to each article. The "Science" category groups together articles that focus on the scientific principles of natural plant stimulation, or on the chemical compounds, the biological agents, etc., that produce this effect, as well as the context of their discovery. A selection of extracts from these articles is shown in Table 7.3.

Media	Quote
Le Figaro (1998)	"His experiments show that plants exposed to caterpillar and aphid attacks at the very beginning of their development are less susceptible later on."
La Tribune (2001)	"Immunostimulation comes from bringing the plant into contact with a molecule that is capable of activating the plant's natural defenses, by spraying it, for example."
Le Télégramme (2002)	"Vaccination with attenuated microbes has been tested with success, in order to fully immunize the plant against cabbage mildew, for example."
Le Monde (2002)	"Over the course of evolution, plants have developed various ways of detecting microbial aggression."
Le Bien Public (2004)	"These elicitors are molecules (of plant or microbial origin) that can act as a real (remote) 'signal' to the plant, which then triggers a natural defense reaction."
Le Point (2004)	"To awaken the vine's defenses, the researcher applies molecules to the vines, notably from seaweed, which simulate aggression."
La Croix (2005)	"It was within these walls that the innate defense mechanisms of plants were discovered."
Le Télégramme (2005)	"Bernard Kloareg, who has been director of the Roscoff biological station for the past two years, is stepping down."
L'Express (2005)	"Other avenues of research are being explored to combat the vine deformation itself or to stimulate the plant's natural defenses."
Le Télégramme (2006)	"On the laboratory side, Bernard Kloareg has associated his name with 'Laminarin'. A substance, naturally present in brown algae, capable of stimulating the immune defenses of plants."
Le Monde (2007)	"There are numerous potential applications of this new tool and researchers are very enthusiastic. These nanoparticles could, for example, be used to vaccinate plants."

Table 7.3. *Quotes from press articles in the "Science" category*

The "Economics (innovation)" category includes articles focusing on SDN-related industrial research, including patent filings. A selection of extracts from these articles is presented in Table 7.4.

Media	Quote
Les Echos (1998)	"The Saint-Malo-based PMI plans to use biotechnology to produce molecules on a large scale that naturally stimulate plants' natural defenses."
Les Echos (1999)	"Goëmar, which devotes 14% of its sales to R&D, has already filed 45 patents in this field."
Le Devoir (2000)	"In its Gaspé laboratory, the company has developed an industrial process for extracting chitin from shrimp shells."
Ouest-France (2004)	"Another innovation is Iodus 40, a defense stimulator derived from the kelp plant, which acts like a vaccine."
Le Point (2005)	"'The company devotes 25% of its sales to research and development, and employs twenty-five researchers,' explains Lionel Labourdette, Administrative and Financial Director."
Ouest-France (2006)	"Based in Saint-Malo since 1972, marine biotechnology company Goëmar, headed by Simon Berteau, develops products for plant health (for agriculture) and human health."
La Tribune (2006)	"In less than ten years, the Goëmar laboratories have won two awards from the French National Institute of Industrial Property (INPI)."
La Tribune (2007)	"Saint-Malo-based company Goëmar has developed a kind of organic plant vaccine called 'Iodus 40' which, when sprayed, helps wheat to mobilize its natural defenses, thus avoiding the need for pesticides."
Le Télégramme (2007)	"Treating plants with algae. This is the main idea of Jacques le Verger, CEO of Osmobio, a company he founded in 1999."

Table 7.4. *Quotes from press articles in the "Economics (innovation)" category*

The "Economics (other)" category groups together articles that focus on the economic aspects of SDN production and marketing. For each article, a quote is presented in Table 7.5.

Media	Quote
Environnement Magazine (2000)	"Goëmar applies for marketing authorization for a vaccination process for plants."
La Tribune (2001)	"He has found the right formula: partnering with an SME and working in total diversity, while also benefiting from funding from the Brittany region."
La Tribune (2001)	"The sea has its markets, but its potential remains insufficiently exploited."
Le Télégramme (2001)	"The partners – scientists, professionals, local authorities – of this public interest group have just renewed their confidence for a further five years."
Le Télégramme (2001)	"The public interest group brings together professional partners such as Cérafel, OBS and Céraflor, scientific partners such as CNRS and UBO, and local authorities such as the regional and general councils, the European Union and the town of Saint-Pol."
La Tribune (2002)	"A few weeks ago, Goëmar, a SME from Brittany, took a full-page advert in *Le Monde* to explain to consumers the benefits of its latest innovation for farmers."
Ouest-France (2005)	"The employees of the Kerplouz experimental station specializing in market gardening are worried about the future of their structure."
Ouest-France (2005)	"For thirty years, Goëmar has been supplying the agricultural sector with seaweed-based bio-stimulants that promote the growth and reproduction of numerous cultivated species, as well as natural plant defense stimulators."
Ouest-France (2006)	"The trophies awarded on Friday in Cancale showcase some of the region's economic flagships. This is the case for the Goëmar company."

Table 7.5. *Quotes from press articles in the "Economics (other)" category*

The "Agriculture" category groups together articles focusing on agricultural practices related to crop protection, or on the promotion of SDNs by agricultural actors, for example, at agricultural fairs. A quote is shown for each article in Table 7.6.

Media	Quote
Ouest-France (2004)	"New techniques such as plant vaccines, a new nitrogen fertilizer, and an agronomic management system were presented."
Le Télégramme (2004)	"The various presenters on site introduced visitors to a plant vaccine that stimulates wheat's natural defenses."
Le Télégramme (2007)	"We explain simple, forgotten or buried techniques that were used in the past. Covering the soil, aromatic plants that promote and stimulate the plants' natural defenses, or simply using potato cooking water to weed!"
Le Devoir (2007)	"Nettle manure stimulates plant strength and natural defenses thanks to the many trace elements found in nettles."
Ouest-France (2007)	"Alternative control methods [...] advocate crop rotations, green manures, disease-resistant varieties, the use of auxiliaries (pest predators), trapping, stimulating the plants' natural defenses..."
Ouest-France (2007)	"In the exhibition aisles, we will be talking about biological protection, natural stimulation of plant defenses or thermal weeding, biodegradable films and packaging, etc."

Table 7.6. *Quotes from press articles in the "Agriculture" category*

The distribution of articles across the four categories is shown in Figure 7.3. Quantitatively, the themes of science and innovation dominate the corpus. The regional press contributes equally to the four categories, while the mainstream press concentrates on the topic of science and the economic press ignores the topic of agriculture.

This focus on science and innovation hand in hand with a universally positive tone towards SDN, with only one article speaking negatively... concerning the low uptake of this control method!

Contrary to the French public's negative opinion of pesticides, SDNs have a positive image, not just because they are not biocidal, toxic or polluting, but also because they are drivers of science and innovation. This original connotation is an integral part of their boundary work.

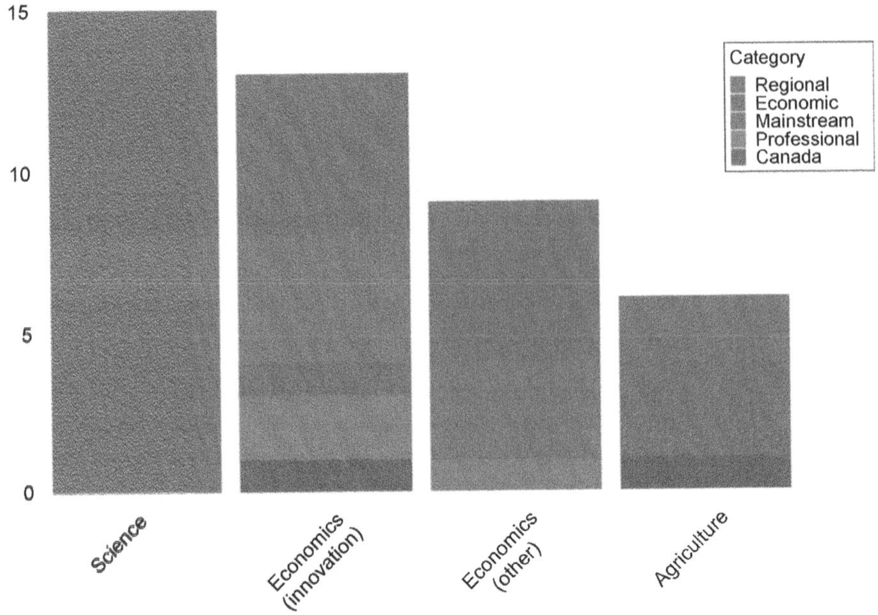

Figure 7.3. *Number of articles on SDNs by theme and category. For a color version of this figure, see: www.iste.co.uk/botero/pesticides.zip*

Furthermore, we also find the previously mentioned argument in the press that SDNs ease the burden of chemical control, by replacing one chemical treatment. Reflecting Goëmar's thoughts on laminarin, *La Tribune* explains that "the use of this technique would halve, even third the use of pesticides, whose residues pollute French waterways"[2], while *Ouest-France* claims that "the farmer reduces his use of fungicides by 25%"[3] and *Le Monde* asserts that "Goëmar does not claim to replace existing products, but to substitute up to 30% of them, at no extra cost"[4]. This cautious stance, far from being unfavorable to SDNs, perfectly realizes their promise.

The SDN sociotechnical network thus avoids public exposure of its struggles (difficulty in controlling its effectiveness in the field, unfavorable marketing procedures, lack of a strong political signal, etc.). Consensual subjects such as

2 Des algues pour protéger les cultures. *La Tribune*, October, 17, 2001.

3 Goëmar invente le vaccin pour blé. *Ouest-France*, November, 19, 2002.

4 Morin, H. (2002). Des molécules tirées des algues brunes stimulent les défenses naturelles des plantes. *Le Monde*, November 21.

innovation and economic dynamics strengthen the network's bonds and help to win over readers, by making certain promises.

7.3.5. *Study of the popular press (1993–2007)*

In addition to the Europresse corpus, we have fortuitously gathered a corpus of six articles, from the popular science and technology press. At first glance, it is an expected result: SDNs are of particular interest to popular science magazines such as *Sciences et avenir* (prior to 1997) and *Pour la science* or *Science & vie* (on two occasions). Unexpectedly, they appear in publications devoted to new technologies and the digital society, such as the US magazine *Wired* or the online magazine *Transfert.net*. Both of these publications are aimed at the tech-savvy part of the general public: the "early adopters" who like to stay abreast of the latest surprising or promising innovations. Once again, SDNs are arousing interest here in terms of innovation and science.

Popular science articles		
Sciences et avenir	Vaccinating plants	No. 557 (July 1993)
Pour la science	Extended wakefulness	No. 255 (January 1999)
Science & vie	Vaccinating plants	No. 994 (July 2000)
Science & vie	We finally know how to vaccinate plants	No. 1081 (October 2007)
Popular web articles		
Wired	A vaccine for plants	https://www.wired.com/2001/09/a-vaccine-for-plants/ (September 4, 2001)
Transfert.net	Beautiful plants, naturally	http://transfert.net/a7225 (September 5, 2001)

Table 7.7. *Popular press articles*

This corpus also highlights the fact that, seven years apart, two articles in *Science & vie* make a very similar observation: "we finally know how to vaccinate plants". In 2000, it was a two-page news brief announcing the marketing of the Messenger® harpine in the United States; in 2007, it was a six-page article on Semafort®, described as "a revolutionary product". The promise of SDNs has not wavered over the period.

7.4. A discursive approach separate to that of biopesticides

The work of linguist Hélène Ledouble offers an interesting point of comparison between the language register of SDNs and that of biopesticides. Let us start by recalling that SDNs and biopesticides are very similar but separate concepts. According to *Larousse agricole*, biopesticides are "biological control agents (auxiliaries, antagonists, entomopathogens, etc.) and active substances produced by some of these agents (*Bacillus thuringiensis* toxin, for example)". They are therefore defined by their biological nature or origin. Catherine Regnault-Roger et al. (2005, p. 851) asked: "can natural plant defense stimulators (SDNs) [...] be considered as biopesticides?", to which she gave a negative answer the following year, discerning between natural substances of plant origin, biopesticides and natural substances of plant origin, SDNs (Regnault-Roger 2006).

While the term "SDN" has become hegemonic in French, the terms "biopesticides" and "biocontrol" have much greater terminological instability, as Hélène Ledouble (2019, 2020) has shown, noting that "different scientific, institutional and legislative perspectives on biopesticides generate an inherent terminological, cognitive and referential complexity" (Ledouble 2020).

We have shown that SDNs are presented as substitutes, as shown in the case for biopesticides in the two excerpts below from the American daily newspaper *The New York Times*, which are analyzed as antonymic relations that contrast biopesticides with chemical pesticides (Ledouble 2020). In this case, however, the substitution is qualitative rather than quantitative:

> It [Bti] is now widely used in place of chemical pesticides (*The New York Times*, 2014).
>
> [...] a pioneer in the development of environmentally safe control agents to replace broad-spectrum chemical pesticides" (*The New York Times*, 2014).

As with SDNs, the discourse on biopesticides is largely positive, with a few occurrences marked by the use of pejorative terms such as "backfire", "controversial", "frightening" and "alarm" (Ledouble 2020):

> [...] most of our customers prefer to deal with a chemical than an animal – it's what they're used to (*The Daily Telegraph* 2014).
>
> Importing tiny insects to tackle Britain's Japanese knotweed problem could easily backfire on us [...] Meddling with nature is always controversial (*The Daily Telegraph* 2010).

> Described as a "voracious invader" with a frightening appetite for other ladybirds [...], the harlequin causes understandable alarm (*The Guardian* 2016).

Lastly, although both our study and that of Hélène Ledouble are intentionally different, and the corpora are not homologous (French corpus over 10 years and English corpus over seven years, respectively), we have applied our coding to the magazines of the biopesticide study, in order to give a more quantitative view (see Figure 7.4). When comparing what is comparable (e.g. the regional press being intentionally absent from Hélène Ledouble's corpus), it appears that the economic press is equal in both corpora, but that the mainstream press reports much more on biopesticides than on SDNs.

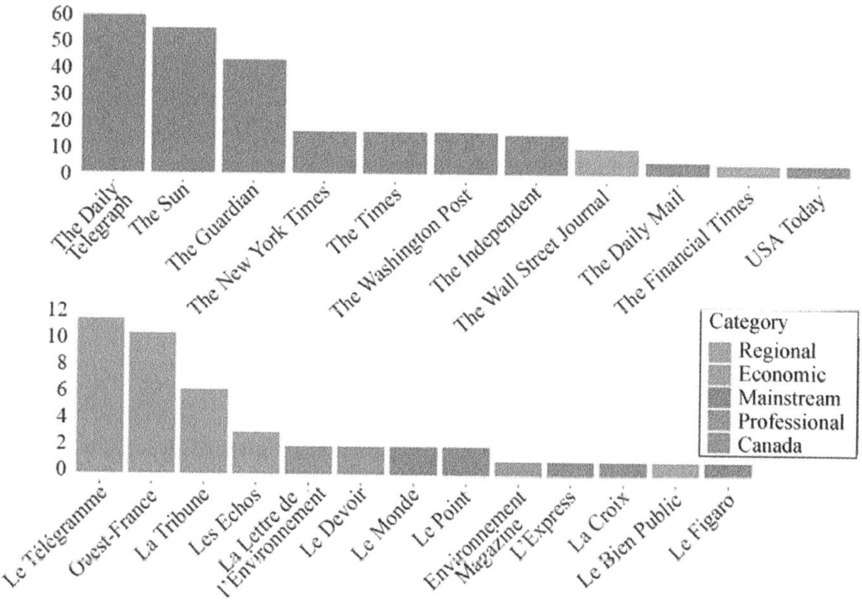

Figure 7.4. *Number of articles on biopesticides (above) and SDNs (below) (see Figure 7.1) by news outlet and category. For a color version of this figure, see: www.iste.co.uk/botero/pesticides.zip*

As SDNs are closer to biopesticides than to any other pesticide, we would expect their media treatment to be relatively similar. Even though the public communication of SDNs and biopesticides plays on the expectations of the public and opinion-formers for nature-friendly farming practices and less productivist agriculture (Fougier 2019), the differences observed reinforce the idea that the discourse on SDNs is actually distinct from that on biopesticides.

7.5. Conclusion

7.5.1. *Discourses to support the SDN sociotechnical network*

The discourses and SDN vocabulary fulfill two main functions: firstly, to maintain the economy of promises, and secondly, to distance themselves from the sociotechnical networks of chemical and biological control. According to Benhamou and Rey (2012), SDNs offer "great promise for the future, because [they] meet growing expectations in terms of environmental and human health protection". To maintain this promise, SDNs must not be reduced to what already exists: they must exist in their own right. Suffering from a perceived lack of effectiveness and irregularity in the field, SDNs were able to rely on a variety of discursive strategies between 1997 and 2007, to keep this promise alive and set themselves apart from other plant protection solutions.

In scientific literature, SDNs are described as a paradigm shift. On the technical and marketing fronts, SDNs adopt brand names that are then confused with other synthetic pesticides, but they also graphically take over product labels to assert their nature as SDNs. In the trade press, the rhetoric of substitution is constantly recurring and is a compelling argument. In the daily press and magazines, SDNs are treated from the journalistic perspective of science, innovation and economics. They have the advantage of novelty and the promise of a more natural agriculture, not only making them desirable to the general public, but to journalists too. This media coverage even sets SDNs apart from biopesticides.

The various areas of communication studied paint a kaleidoscopic picture of the SDN network, bringing together communities of researchers, industrialists, public authorities and journalists (farmers are conspicuously absent) around a common repertoire that fabricates the "SDN world" we are a part of. There is however one exception: in the trade press, as in technical and marketing documentation, agrochemical multinational companies do not join the sociotechnical network, in stark contrast to the development of the electric car in the 1970s, where the French giant EDF "distributes the roles, binds together these actors and shows what each must do to adapt to the scientific and technical evolutions foreseen" (Callon 1981, p. 394). This is not the case with the SDNs. Instead, the collective has failed to win over the dominant actors in the agricultural sector. In 2010, the *Réseau mixte technologique* (Mixed technology network (RMT)) Elicitra, accredited by the French Ministry of Agriculture, which brought together around 30 consular, scientific, technical and industry actors, was even set up without the multinational companies. Its major ambition was to accelerate the development of SDNs by decompartmentalizing and coordinating the work carried out by each actor, for the benefit of the agricultural sectors.

7.5.2. *A recent trend marked by the rise of biocontrol*

It has to be said that SDNs have not yet established themselves in the field, even if they benefit from a dynamic biocontrol sector, the new category in which they are included. Therefore, while the market for chemical pesticides was expected to grow by just 3% a year between 2012 and 2020, the market for biocontrol solutions was set to increase by 15% a year to reach 8% of crop protection sales by 2020 (Chomienne et al. 2017). In the end, it exceeded 12% of the market (IBMA France 2021). These economic projections are especially favorable to agrochemical multinational companies: in INRAE's *Sesame* magazine, the marketing director of Bioline AgroSciences-group InVivo warned that:

> All of the companies that offered, or could offer, these types of solutions requiring registration have been bought out, or will be bought out, by the major phytosanitary groups – Bayer, BASF, Syngenta and others (Gillot and Péan 2018).

A report commissioned by the *Centre d'études et de prospective du ministère de l'Agriculture*[5] (Faessel et al. 2014, p. 104) thus reveals five acquisitions of companies that produced SDNs between 2012 and 2014.

From a regulatory point of view, SDNs benefit from the depreciation for low-risk active substances set out in Regulation 1107/2009 of the European Parliament, and of the Council of October 21, 2009, concerning the release of plant protection products on the market. The Law of October 13, 2014, on the future of agriculture, food and forestry includes measures to promote the marketing of biocontrol products, notably through an accelerated assessment and authorization procedure, as well as to facilitate their use. SDNs are also among the biocontrol products that benefit from a reduced tax under the March 9, 2016, order, setting the rate of the sales tax of plant protection products.

One unexpected outcome remains to be mentioned: while the terminological stability of SDNs was their strength:

> The INDRES network (for INduction De RESistance), which is made up of some twenty French scientists, [has] proposed that the term *SDP* (for *stimulateur de défense des plantes*: plant defense stimulator) replace the term *SDN*, in order to include synthetic products (Benhamou and Rey 2012).

The INDRES network is "also working to limit the marketing of empirical products for which no scientific data is available", even though "no SDN

5 Center for Studies and Prospective.

registrations [have] been issued in the last five years", which could explain this eagerness to regulate the sector (Benhamou and Rey 2012). A new investigation into the vocabulary could be conducted to document and monitor this terminological development.

7.6. References

Attruia, F. (2020). Les discours de l'Union européenne sur la biodiversité : une analyse des registres communicationnels. *Les carnets du Cediscor*, 15, 49–63.

Benhamou, N. and Rey, P. (2012). Stimulateurs des défenses naturelles des plantes : une nouvelle stratégie phytosanitaire dans un contexte d'écoproduction durable. II. Intérêt des SDN en protection des cultures. *Phytoprotection*, 92(1), 24–35.

Berelson, B. (1952). *Content Analysis in Communication Research*. Free Press, New York.

Blanchard, A. (2016). From one community to many: How novel objects in the crop protection field reveal epistemic boundaries. *Social Epistemology*, 30(5–6), 680–691.

Blanchard, A. (2018a). Les stimulateurs des défenses naturelles des plantes (SDN). Histoire d'une innovation phytosanitaire (1977–2007). *Cahiers COSTECH – cahiers connaissance, organisation et systèmes techniques*, 1 [Online]. Available at: https://hal.science/hal-01633345v2..

Blanchard, A. (2018b). Chronologie des dépôts de brevets relatifs au Bion®. doi: 10.6084/m9.figshare.7007537.v2 [Accessed August 22, 2022].

Bouron, H., Mutschler, J.-M., Decoin, M. (1998). L'évolution de la protection des cultures. *Phytoma – La défense des végétaux*, 506, 13–15.

Callon, M. (1981). Pour une sociologie des controverses technologiques. *Fundamenta Scientiæ*, 2(3/4), 381–399.

Callon, M. (1986). Éléments pour une sociologie de la traduction : la domestication des coquilles St-Jacques et des marins pêcheurs dans la baie de St. Brieuc. *L'Année sociologique*, 36, 169–208.

Callon, M. and Law, J. (1989). La protohistoire d'un laboratoire. In *La Science et ses réseaux*, Callon, M. (ed.). La Découverte/Conseil de l'Europe/ UNESCO, Paris.

Chomienne, J.-P., Dutartre, S., Larguier, M., Pinçonnet, D., Tessier, R. (2017). Les produits de biocontrôle pour la protection des cultures. Report, Conseil général de l'alimentation de l'agriculture et des espaces ruraux, Paris.

Cole, D.L. (2008). Book review: D. Walters, A. Newton and G. Lyon, induced resistance for plant defence. *Crop Protection*, 27(3–5), 882.

Edreva, A. (2004). A novel strategy for plant protection: Induced resistance. *Journal of Cell and Molecular Biology*, 3(2), 61–69.

Faessel, L., Gomy, C., Nassr, N., Tostivint, C., Hipper, C., Dechanteloup, A. (2014). Produits de stimulation en agriculture visant à améliorer les fonctionnalités biologiques des sols et des plantes – étude des connaissances disponibles et recommandations stratégiques. Report, BIO by Deloitte and RITTMO Agroenvironnement, Paris.

Férez, J.-M., Duchon-Doris, J., Decoin, M. (2008). Les trois domaines du *Bacillus thuringiensis*. *Phytoma – La défense des végétaux*, 613, 10–13.

Fèvre-Pernet, C. and Roché, M. (2005). Quel traitement lexicographique de l'onomastique commerciale ? Pour une distinction Nom de marque/Nom de produit. *Corela*, HS-2. doi: 10.4000/corela.1198.

Fixari, D. and Hatchuel, A. (1998). Les méthodes de lutte contre la pyrale du maïs. In *Les chercheurs et l'innovation : regards sur les pratiques de l'INRA*. INRA Éditions, Paris.

Fougier, E. (2019). L'hostilité des acteurs de la transition écologique à l'encontre des agriculteurs. *Paysans & société*, 375(3), 32–38.

Fourche, R. (2004). Contribution à l'histoire de la protection phytosanitaire dans l'agriculture française (1880-1970). PhD Thesis, Université Lumière, Lyon.

Fournier, J. (2006). Naissances de la protection chimique des cultures. *L'Actualité Chimique*, 298, 43–53.

Gillot, L. and Péan, V. (2018). Biocontrôle : gare aux confusions textuelles. *Sesame*, 3, 46–49.

IBMA France (2021). Le biocontrôle poursuit sa progression en 2020. Press Release, Les Culturales. Available at: https://www.ibmafrance.com/wp-content/uploads/2021/06/210615_Dossier_Presse_IBMA_France.pdf [Accessed 3 February 2023].

Joly, P.-B. and Lemarié, S. (2002). The technological trajectories of the agrochemical industry: Change and continuity. *Science and Public Policy*, 29(4), 259–266.

Jourdheuil, P., Grison, P., Fraval, A. (1991). La lutte biologique : un aperçu historique. *Le Courrier de la cellule environnement*, 15, 37–60.

Kessmann, H., Staub, T., Hofmann, C., Maetzke, T., Herzog, J., Ward, E., Uknes, S., Ryals, J. (1994). Induction of systemic acquired disease resistance in plants by chemicals. *Annual Review of Phytopathology*, 32, 439–459.

Kidd, H. (2002). Insect pests – Crumbling defences and new approaches. *Pesticide Outlook*, 13, 201–203.

Klarzynski, O. and Fritig, B. (2001). Stimulation des défenses naturelles des plantes. *Comptes rendus de l'académie des sciences. Série 3 : sciences de la vie*, 324(10), 953–963.

Klarzynski, O., Descamps, V., Plesse, B., Yvin, J., Kloareg, B., Fritig, B. (2003). Sulfated fucan oligosaccharides elicit defense responses in tobacco and local and systemic resistance against tobacco mosaic virus. *Molecular Plant-Microbe Interactions*, 16(2), 115–122.

Kogan, M. (1998). Integrated pest management: Historical perspectives and contemporary developments. *Annual Review of Entomology*, 43, 243–270.

Krieg-Planque, A. (2010). La formule "développement durable" : un opérateur de neutralisation de la conflictualité. *Langage et société*, 134(4), 5–29.

Kuhn, T.S. (1983). *La structure des révolutions scientifiques*, 2nd edition. Flammarion, Paris.

Kunz, W., Schurter, R., Maetzke, T. (1997). The chemistry of benzothiadiazole plant activators. *Pesticide Science*, 50(4), 275–282.

Latour, B. (1997). *Nous n'avons jamais été modernes. Essai d'anthropologie symétrique*, 2nd edition. La Découverte, Paris.

Leadbeater, A. and Staub, T. (2007). Exploitation of induced resistance: A commercial perspective. In *Induced Resistance for Plant Defence: A Sustainable Approach to Crop Protection*, Walters, D., Newton, A.C., Lyon, G.D. (eds). Blackwell Publishing, Oxford.

Leblanc, B. and Bilodeau, C. (2007). Les noms de marques de médicaments : points de repères linguistiques et onomastiques. In *La chaîne des médicaments : perspectives pluridisciplinaires*, Lévy, J. and Garnier, C. (eds). Presses de l'Université du Québec, Quebec.

Ledouble, H. (2019). Vulgarisation scientifique et médiatisation de la science : instabilité terminologique dans le domaine de la lutte biologique. *Terminology*, 25(1), 60–92.

Ledouble, H. (2020). Term circulation and conceptual instability in the mediation of science: Binary framing of the notions of biological versus chemical pesticides. *Discourse & Communication*, 14, 466–488.

Lemarié, S., Jorge, I., Joly, P.-B. (2001). PITA Project Annex D3: SMEs in the French agrochemicals, seeds and plant biotechnology industries. Report, INRA – SERD, Paris. Available at: http://technology.open.ac.uk/cts/pita/AnnD3-SMEs-FR.pdf [Accessed August 22, 2022].

Lucas, J.A. (1999). Plant immunisation: From myth to SAR. *Pesticide Science*, 55(2), 193–196.

Lyon, G.D. (2007). Agents that can elicit induced resistance. In *Induced Resistance for Plant Defence: A Sustainable Approach to Crop Protection*, Walters, D., Newton, A.C., Lyon, G.D. (eds). Blackwell Publishing, Oxford.

Lyon, G.D. and Newton, A.C. (1997). Do resistance elicitors offer new opportunities in integrated disease control strategies? *Plant Pathology*, 46, 636–641.

Lyon, G.D. and Newton, A.C. (1999). Implementation of elicitor-mediated induced resistance in agriculture. In *Induced Plant Defences Against Pathogens and Herbivores*, Agrawal, A.A., Tuzun, S., Bent, E. (eds). APS Press, St. Paul.

Maingueneau, D. (2014). *Discours et analyse du discours*. Armand Colin, Paris.

Mortureux, M.-F. (1984). La dénomination, approche socio-linguistique. *Langages*, 76, 95–112.

Oostendorp, M., Kunz, W., Dietrich, B., Staub, T. (2001). Induced disease resistance in plants by chemicals. *European Journal of Plant Pathology*, 107(1), 19–28.

Pajot, E., Maurice, S., Guerrand, J., Chirapongsatonkul, N., de Ruffray, P., Kauffmann, S., Maxant, F.-X., du Mérac, H. (2007). Sur tabac, fraise et vigne, travaux sur un fertilisant pouvant stimuler des défenses naturelles des plantes. *Phytoma – La défense des végétaux*, 603, 38–41.

Pellissier, F. (2021). Tuer les pestes pour protéger les cultures : sociohistoire de l'administration des pesticides en France. PhD Thesis, Université Gustave Eiffel, Marne-la-Vallée.

Philogène, B.J.R., Fabres, G., Regnault-Roger, C. (2005). Protection des cultures, environnement et développement durable : enjeux pour le XXIe siècle. In *Enjeux phytosanitaires pour l'agriculture et l'environnement*, Regnault-Roger, C. (ed.). Lavoisier, Paris.

Regnault-Roger, C. (2006). Les substances naturelles d'origine végétale. Qu'elles soient biopesticides ou éliciteurs (SDN), quelles sont leurs perspectives dans la protection des cultures ? *Phytoma*, 591, 14–18.

Regnault-Roger, C., Silvy, C., Alabouvette, C. (2005). Biopesticides : réalités et perspectives commerciales. In *Enjeux phytosanitaires pour l'agriculture et l'environnement*, Regnault-Roger, C. (ed.). Lavoisier, Paris.

Rossignol, Y., Rambach, O., Petit, M., Ruess, W.S. (1997). L'acibenzolar-S-methyl : une nouvelle catégorie de produits pour la protection des cultures. In *5e conférence internationale sur les maladies des plantes*. Association française de protection des plantes, Tours.

Wenger, E. (1999). *Communities of Practice: Learning, Meaning and Identity*. Cambridge University Press, Cambridge.

Yacoub, P. (2021). Des prescripteurs à la croisée des chemins : le marché du conseil agricole face à la séparation des activités de conseil et de vente de pesticides. MSc Thesis, Institut d'études politiques, Paris.

8

Circulation of Discourses and Counter-discourses about Pesticides on Social Networks

8.1. Introduction

For several decades now, the question of the dangerousness of pesticides has been making more or less high-profile forays into public debate. While a fair number of studies and legal positions have been communicated in several countries around the world (Jouzel 2019), the complexity of the subject itself creates a massive production of discourses and counter-discourses, similar to the issue regarding the difference between chemical and biological pesticides (Ledouble 2020). Discourses and counter-discourses about pesticides seem to vary. Indeed, from neonicotinoids (Collet and Charreton 2017) to glyphosates (Campion 2019), public media controversies have given rise to a wide variety of narratives that have largely influenced the way individuals represent the substances used in agriculture.

The aim of this chapter is to build on the "culture of commenting on comments" (Wagener 2018) which occurs within social networks through what is known as hypernarrativity (Wagener 2020). To this end, we have made up a corpus to access these representations within discourses (Baker 2006), while considering the specific aspects of discourses related to the environment and ecology (Fracchiolla 2019). This corpus gives rise to a lexicometric analysis of co-occurrences (Bendinelli 2011; Martinez 2012), in order to map out speaker representations (Barbazan 2011), as well as their stance in relation to societal issues related to pesticides.

Chapter written by Albin WAGENER.

From this point of view, it is indeed the comments, and not the publications themselves, that constitute the material on which the corpus is built. The corpus is drawn from the social networks Facebook, YouTube and Reddit, and to analyze it, we use digital tools both to compile it (notably Crowdtangle and Facepager) and to analyze it (more specifically, thanks to Iramuteq).

Within this context, Chapter 8 is structured as follows:

– a theoretical framework, based on discourse analysis applied to the corpus (section 8.2);

– the corpus construction methodology (section 8.3);

– an analysis of the results obtained from the digital study of the corpus (section 8.4);

– and lastly, the interpretation of these results (section 8.5).

This work also aims to provide an overview of the discourses within social networks, as post-digital tools (Andersen et al. 2014). Through a digital analysis of these productions, the objective is to understand how the term "pesticides" (and some of its associated terms, such as "neonicotinoids" or "glyphosate") are used in the public sphere, in order to better grasp its linguistic particularities and symbolic representations, which reflect a number of contemporary social issues around ecology, food and public health.

8.2. A discursive analysis of corpora

The discursive analysis of corpora is a branch of discourse analysis, which aims to understand the articulation of arguments within language productions (Amossy 2011), the way in which these arguments sustainably impact the social representations that circulate in the public space (Fairclough 1992), the preconceptions at work in these language productions (Paveau 2006), and the way in which all of these aspects are embodied within the media space itself (Moirand 2007). Discourse analysis thus makes it possible to suggest links with the study of the construction and reception of communication phenomena (Charaudeau 2007), as well as with the circulation of information within societies (Calabrese 2014).

First of all, we would like to emphasize that our study is part of what may be called a sociolinguistic and systemic analysis of discourse, i.e. an analysis that allows us to isolate and study the representations within language and semiotics (thus also taking non-linguistic approaches into account). It is thus possible to link these formations to schools of thought and social practices, using a methodology that crosses several analytical choices. This stance calls for a specific definition of the notion of discourse:

> [Discourse] is any language phenomenon (therefore linguistic, but not exclusively so) whose purpose is the construction, exchange and transformation of a social meaning with a sense of structure, potentially politically significant, and necessarily rooted in essential intersubjectivity, whether it be intentional or not, in other words, which is produced and received by subjects, who may express themselves individually or collectively, about shareable purposes (Wagener 2019, p. 39).

This definition of discourse obviously, on the contrary, has an impact on the notion of counter-discourse being accepted. By clearly positioning discourses in their social environment, we can study them through their lexical inputs (Née and Veniard 2012), so as to gain access to the representations they house and express. It is these representational spaces, as defined by Marion Bendinelli through her work on the analysis of presidential debates in the United States, that we can access through the study of the corpus proposed in the present work:

> Representational spaces provide an original key to reading underlying statements, since they enable us to "see" the world that the speaker constructs and the relationships he or she maintains with the elements that make it up. In so doing, they offer the possibility of identifying some of the knowledge required for interpretation (Bendinelli 2011, p. 110).

As a result, the study of the corpus through the use of lexical items emphasizes their semantic charge. In other words, the choice of words is never separate from the social dynamics of meaning, which has notable effects on the expression of arguments within discourse, as well as on the circulation of the latter.

Isolated in this way, semantic elements are perceived as being connected and exchanging information (Barbazan 2011) within interdiscursive environments (Garric and Longhi 2013), insofar as they can be perceived as places where a wide variety of discourses and counter-discourses intersect, clash and are projected. In order to study these elements, we have chosen to build a corpus which can provide information about the circulating discourses (Baker 2006): this structuring, within the digital media space (Rouquette 2016; Reyna et al. 2018), makes it possible to indicate the scope of certain lexemes. In other words, the use of certain words over others is likely to cause a chain of discursive reactions and productions, such as the ripples caused by a pebble thrown into water. Access to representations is thus achieved through a linguistic corpus study, to echo the work of Paul Baker:

> Corpus linguistics, in addition to helping to reduce bias, is a useful way of approaching discourse analysis, because of the incremental effect of discourse. One of the most important ways in which discourses are circulated and reinforced in society is through the use of language, and the mission of discourse analysts is to reveal how language is used, often in rather subtle ways, in order to reveal underlying discourses […]. Thus, a simple word, phrase or grammatical construction can in itself suggest the existence of discourse […]. And this is where corpora come in handy. An association between two words, repeatedly produced in natural language, is far more relevant proof of underlying hegemonic discourse, made explicit through lexical collocation, than a simple case (Baker 2006, p. 13).

Here, the approach of the corpus study begins with an initial study of the analysis of co-occurrences in the corpus; i.e. the positioning of terms in relation to one another, and the frequency of a few of these lexical similarities. This tool-based analysis has been produced thanks to seminal work carried out over more than 30 years in "French-styled" discourse analysis, which has worked extensively on co-occurrence phenomena (Tournier 1985; Martinez 2012), analysis methodology (Reinert 1990) and the development of digital tools (Marchand 1998). It is in this continuity, both analytical and critical, that we establish our work.

While the aim of this text is obviously to understand the way in which discourse circulates on social networks, particularly through a position that combines discourse study and the use of lexicometric corpus analysis tools, it should also be noted that the whole of this controversy is also influenced by its speaking environment; i.e. by the digital devices which enable web users to comment under videos and articles. Through the extraction of comments built up into a corpus, the analysis provides access to a network of narratives (Benhabib 2002) that individuals place themselves into, and from which they can also choose to leave. Individuals thus interact within a hypernarrative environment (Wagener 2020), already influenced by previous discourses on environmental and ecological controversies (Alexander 2009; Biros 2014), and are shaped by their own experience of using the Internet and social networks:

> The entire Web offers an experience of information that has no beginning, no middle, no end, and is always infinite and impossible to finish, insofar as social networking sites, video games, tweets and web pages weave into another to create a ubiquitous environment of information. It is through this environment that we travel, bouncing from one disconnected nugget of information to the next (Rose 2012, p. 99)[1].

1 Translation by the author.

8.3. Corpus and methodology

As previously mentioned, we chose to build a corpus from social networks in order to identify the way in which pesticide-related themes were addressed from the perspective of discourse circulation. The corpus studied in this article is made up of comments that have been extracted from various social network publications. These publications are selected according to their engagement rate; this can be defined as the way in which publications acquire a high degree of visibility and virality by combining the number of reactions (such as *likes* on Facebook) and reposts on other social networking platforms from Internet users (Hwong et al. 2017). To gain an insight into the engagement rate of these publications, we used the CrowdTangle[2] tool, which maps the most engaging publications over a given period, based on keywords entered into the search engine. In other words, this is a tool for what is known as *social listening*, i.e. observing what is circulating on social networks and the performance of publications (Stewart and Arnold 2018).

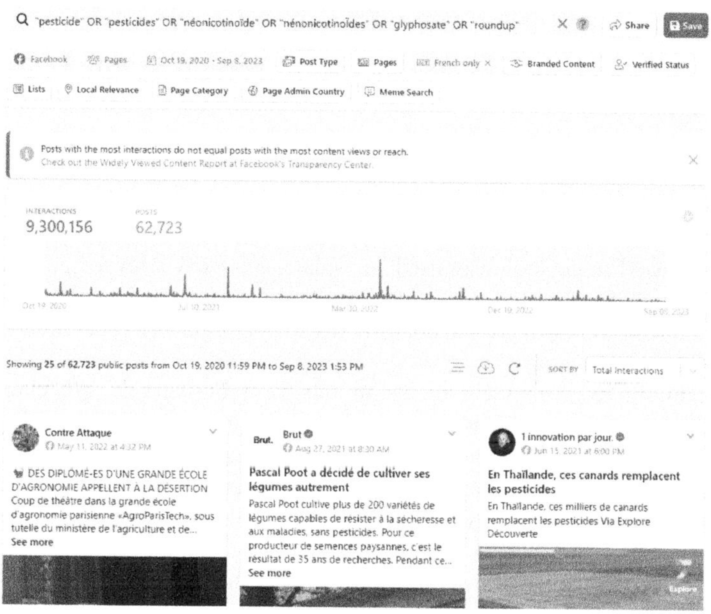

Figure 8.1. *Screenshot of CrowdTangle digital tool*

To obtain relevant results, we used a query that includes several keywords which are particularly effective in obtaining content tailored to our work's subject: ("pesticides" OR "pesticide" OR "neonicotinoid" OR "neonicotinoids" OR

2 See: www.crowdtangle.com/ [Accessed May 25, 2023].

"glyphosate" OR "roundup"). This choice of lexemes was made in order to focus the search on media-related terms that are specifically cited in discussions, debates and controversies around these subjects, and which are used both in publications and in the social media keyword repertoire (one of the bases of these so-called "Boolean queries" (Frants et al. 1999)). This query was applied over a period running from October 1, 2020 to October 1, 2021, in order to achieve a sufficiently large representation over 12 months, while also staying within realm of discursive news. The purpose of this query was to obtain publications that offered a significant number of comments; indeed, it is not the media productions themselves which interest us here, but the way in which individuals react to and comment on them, thus enabling a wide diversity of discourses and counter-discourses. We were thus able to acquire 59 comment threads reacting to 59 publications, broken down as follows:

– Facebook (19 publications out of 20, as the comments for one of them could not be extracted), on pages such as *Brut*, *France 5*, *Hugo Clément*, *Le Parisien*, *Arte*, *Greenpeace* or *Lucie Lucas*, which combine informative publications with the accounts of influencers or activist organizations.

– Reddit (20 publications), all from French pages (except two from Quebec pages), which relay either articles published in the press or scientific articles.

– YouTube (20 videos), with pages from *Le Monde*, *Arte*, *Brut*, *Konbini*, *Le Parisien*, *Greenletter Club* and *Temps Présent*, as well as personal videos from, for example, a Loiret farmer or Pierre Girard.

The CrowdTangle tool was used to isolate the most relevant publications on Facebook and Reddit; however, for YouTube (unfortunately absent from the CrowdTangle search results), the platform's search engine was used directly.

In addition, to extract comments in the form of datasets, we chose to use Facepager[3], an open-source tool available on GitHub and developed by German researchers. Using APIs (application programming interfaces), it is possible to extract a wide variety of content and data from several websites, provided we have an account that gives us access to them.

Thanks to Facepager, it is possible to extract and compile comments through database files, which can then be structured into a corpus and analyzed using traditional lexicometric analysis tools.

To analyze these comment sets, we chose the Iramuteq[4] tool, which has been used for many years in both the scientific and professional worlds.

3 See: www.github.com/strohne/Facepager.

4 See: www.iramuteq.org/.

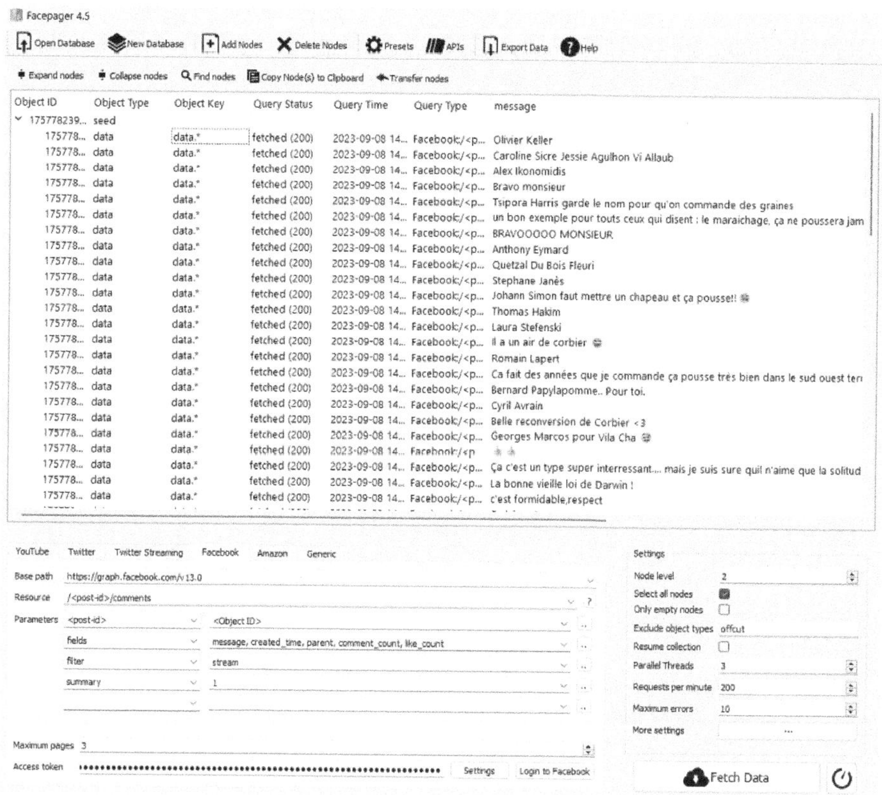

Figure 8.2. *Screenshot of the Facepager digital tool*

To enable Iramuteq to access and analyze the lexical content of these comments, all of the data is compiled and encoded in a text file. The first results proposed by the software give the following statistics:

– 59 comment threads;

– approximately 16,800 comments for Facebook, 2,300 for YouTube and 150 for Reddit;

– 389,674 occurrences (or words);

– 22,877 occurrences used regularly in the corpus;

– 12,777 hapax (words used only once).

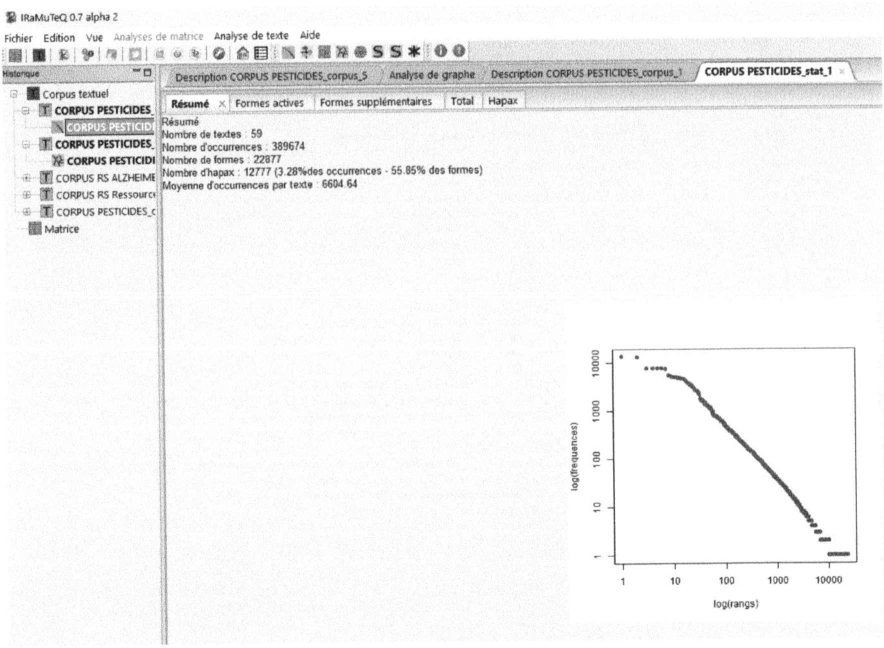

Figure 8.3. *Screenshot of the Iramuteq digital tool. For a color version of this figure, see www.iste.co.uk/botero/pesticides.zip*

The first point to note here is that the wide disparity in comments between the three social networks can be explained by the fact that, generally speaking, conversations are more fruitful on Facebook than on YouTube, particularly in terms of the exchange of comments. As for Reddit, this smaller platform offers corpus elements that make it possible to isolate a specific community. The latter, as we shall see, sees pesticides as a technological advance, enabling agriculture to feed a large population. In any case, with these clarifications in place, Iramuteq can isolate the lexical forms that are most frequently used in this corpus, as well as calculate the co-occurrence frequencies between terms; in other words, the most frequent similarities between words in the corpus, while keeping in mind that the proximity of certain terms determines emerging social representations (Martinez 2012).

8.4. Analysis results

The first analysis results offered by Iramuteq allow us to visualize the most frequent (or the most repeated) lexical occurrences in the corpus, through a word cloud; that is a classic way of presenting the data, but one that is essential for obtaining an initial lexicometric map of the corpus.

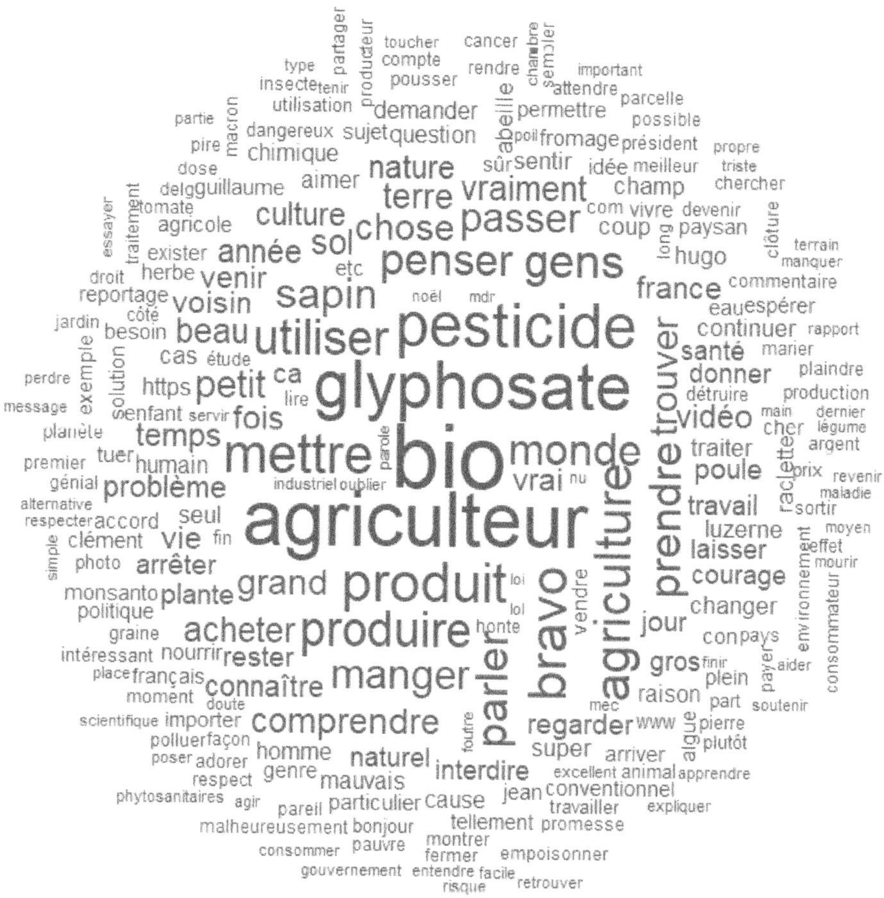

Figure 8.4. *Word cloud of the Iramuteq corpus*

This first visualization already offers some interesting information on the link made in the comments between terms such as pesticides, agriculture, production and organic. The occurrence of verbs such as "produce" or "eat" offers an immediate contextualization of the way in which Internet users seem to appropriate these issues, at least within the three social networks studied. This first corpus extraction obviously needs to be supplemented by more detailed analyses.

A second option suggested by Iramuteq is to visualize the links between the most representative occurrences in the corpus, thus locating lexical co-occurrences within a wider textual environment and also providing an initial representation of the semantic and thematic links that structure the corpus. This option, known as similarity analysis in the software, produces the image shown in Figure 8.5.

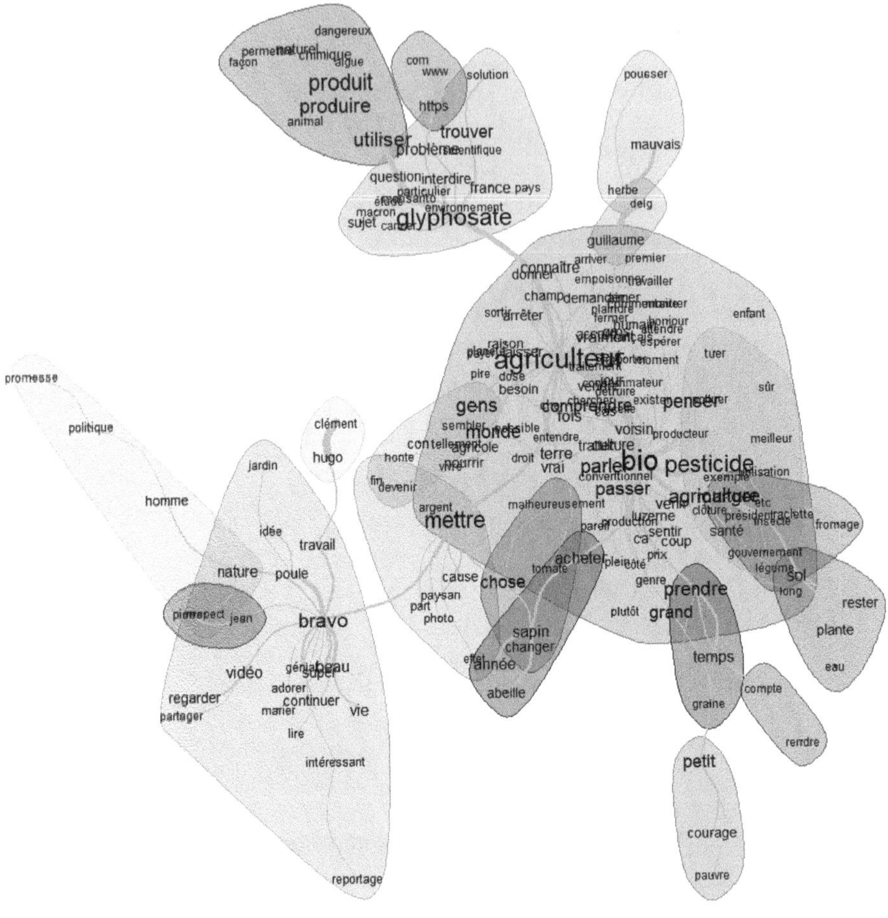

Figure 8.5. *Similarity analysis of the Iramuteq corpus. For a color version of this figure, see www.iste.co.uk/botero/pesticides.zip*

We can distinguish several features, notably the creation of meaningful sets of words:

– A first set is linked to agricultural production itself (in the center-right of the visualization), with terms such as "farmer", "organic", "pesticide" or "agriculture".

– A second set is linked to the controversy and issues surrounding the use of glyphosate (near the top), particularly in relation to agricultural production issues.

– Lastly, a final set (to the bottom-left of the visualization) highlights the comments made by Internet users in relation to content, reflecting both the strong interactional aspect of the corpus and reactions to investigative reporting or news videos, which give rise to comments.

This initial visualization obviously allows us to grasp other nuances but, above all, it provides clues on how to understand the use of certain terms over others, as well as the links between sets of occurrences.

The next step is to take these clues into account in the analysis, and obtain a more detailed look at the corpus, according to the themes.

These are analyzed by Iramuteq using the Reinert method (Reinert 1990), enabling a breakdown of the corpus according to the major themes addressed. This is particularly effective alongside the similarity analysis. This analysis, based on parameters that can be adapted, provides a clear picture of the themes addressed in the corpus, as well as the lexical occurrences which are linked to them.

In our corpus, Iramuteq isolates five thematic classes, which we describe below (from left to right in Figure 8.6):

– class 3 ('classe 3' in Figure 8.6): a very strong social interaction around the investigative and informative work of the various publications, which also highlights the extent to which social networks are interaction-intensive tools;

– class 4 ('classe 4' in Figure 8.6): a theme that illustrates the issues associated with being close to land sprayed with pesticides, and therefore also rural cohabitation with farmers who practice this type of production;

– class 2 ('classe 2' in Figure 8.6): a broader theme, dealing with the impact of pesticides on nature;

– class 1 ('classe 1' in Figure 8.6): a class dedicated to pesticides as chemical products, offering food for thought, as well as questions about their composition and effects;

– class 5 ('classe 5' in Figure 8.6): a final class focusing on the impact on consumption and food, with a strong representation of controversy related to the discovery of pesticide traces on the rind of certain raclette cheeses.

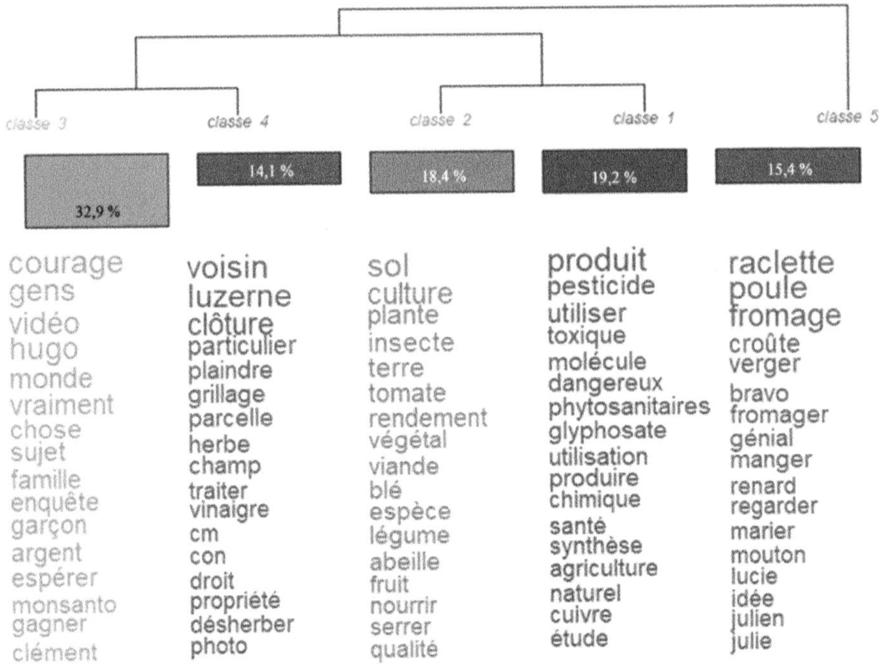

Figure 8.6. *Dendrogram analysis of the Iramuteq corpus. For a color version of this figure, see www.iste.co.uk/botero/pesticides.zip*

These five thematic classes give clear indications of the way in which polarizing discourses within comments produce content: in addition to the interactional aspect in social networks and reactions to investigative and news documentaries, there is a social aspect (neighboring with farmers who spray pesticides), an environmental aspect (effects on nature), a food aspect and a purely scientific aspect (around the chemical composition of pesticides).

These thematic classes can be represented in a separate diagram, in order to highlight the distance or proximity between certain subjects. This is what Iramuteq offers, thanks to correspondence factor analysis (CFA).

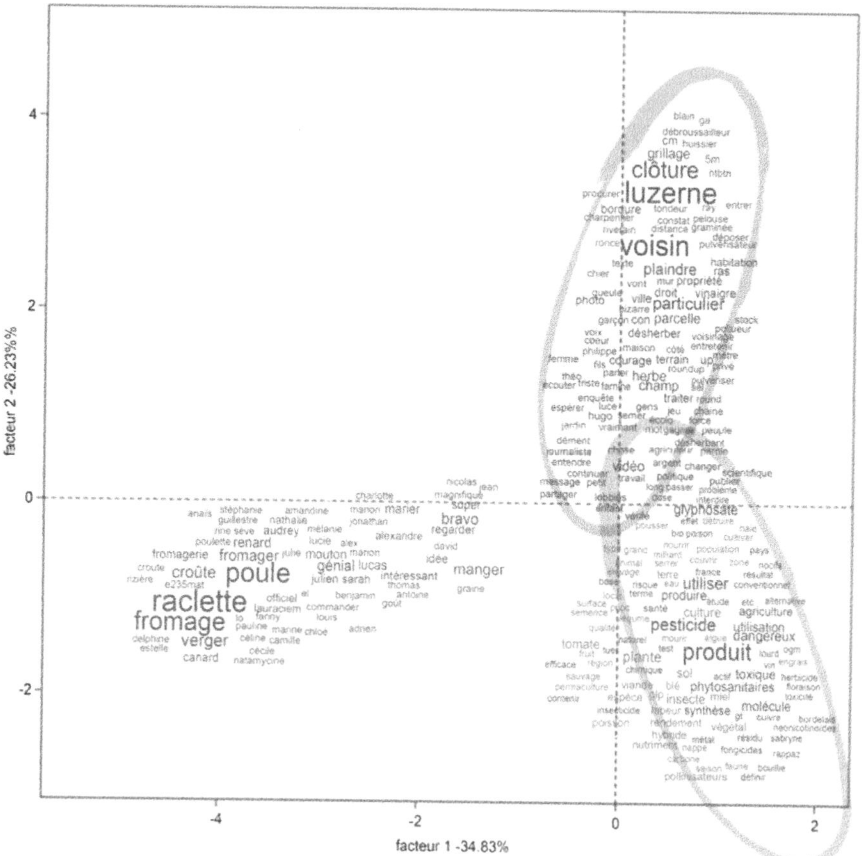

Figure 8.7. *Correspondence factor analysis (CFA) of the Iramuteq corpus. For a color version of this figure, see www.iste.co.uk/botero/pesticides.zip*

Figure 8.7 shows that the thematic classes have specific relationships with one another, which highlights the closeness of certain discussions within the comments:

– To the bottom-right of this CFA, class 2 (effects on nature) and class 1 (synthetic nature of pesticides) are interrelated, highlighting an opposition between the "natural" and "synthetic" aspects, and more broadly, human intervention on environments that are influenced or modified by the products we inject into them.

– To the top-right of the visualization, class 4 (proximity to farmers) and class 3 (reactions to investigations and information) are close to one another, with class 3 at the center of the CFA: this feature also shows individuals' sensitivity to information about pesticides and, beyond the issue of public health, the logics of close exposure to these substances, for example, in rural or peri-urban areas.

– Lastly, on the left side of the visualization, class 5 (consumption and food) seems further removed from the others, which shows how food is viewed in terms of pesticide-related controversies.

What is surprising here is the distance between discourse on food and its effects on health, on the one hand, and conversations about the composition of pesticides and their effects on nature, on the other hand; it would seem that interactions within social networks more easily link the harmful effects of pesticides to the direct natural environment, rather than to the food ingested. This specificity is likely significant, and perhaps reflects both the symbolic weight of food (and even gastronomy, given the French cultural aspect of the corpus), at the very least in terms of tasting and pleasure, where production in the direct natural environment is instead related to the situation of agricultural production as an artisanal or industrial process.

With this in mind, it is also important to observe the intricacies of different conversations within digital environments, based on the specific elements that make up the corpus. Therefore, when encoding the corpus, it is possible to indicate variables that qualify the sets of comments – depending on, for example, the subject of the publication being commented on or the social network of publication – which then enables the analysis to offer particularly instructive points of comparison. This specific feature enables Iramuteq to suggest a CFA of these variables, which of course takes up the specific themes, while also highlighting certain particularities.

We can already see that social networks are more or less represented according to the thematic conversations, which enriches our understanding of the mapping of the corpus:

– For example, Facebook seems to be better represented in class 5 discussions (food and consumption), notably due to the controversy surrounding raclette cheese and the traces of pesticides found in the crusts of certain brands.

– As for YouTube, it is class 3 (interactions around investigation) that seems to be particularly highlighted, which explains the interest of videos in the transmission of information and Internet users' attachment to this format.

– Lastly, and to no surprise, Reddit is represented in class 1 discussions (pesticide composition), as this network often brings scientists and engineers together on a wide range of discourse subjects.

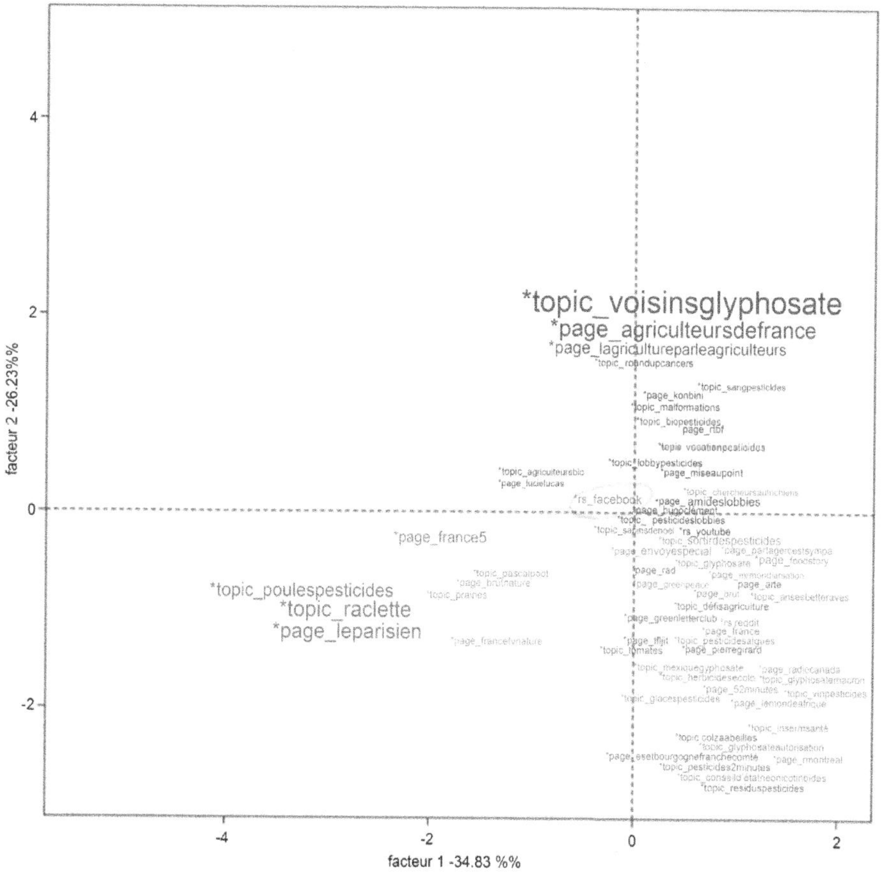

Figure 8.8. *Correspondence factor analysis (CFA) of the Iramuteq corpus variables. For a color version of this figure, see www.iste.co.uk/botero/pesticides.zip*

There are also specifics according to the pages that published the articles (*Le Parisien* on Facebook, for example, or Konbini on YouTube), as well as according to subjects (or topics) that trigger a high rate of engagement. For example, the CFA variable of the corpus shows that reactions to information, such as that materialized within class 3, focus particularly on the subjects of biopesticides, deformities, cancers caused by Roundup, an Élise Lucet report or a video on the lobbyist structure of certain pesticide manufacturers. On the contrary, in class 1 (where Reddit is overrepresented), pages such as those of Greenpeace, *Brut*, *Envoyé Spécial* or *Le Monde* offer content that seems to encourage Internet users to engage in discourse and counter-discourse on the chemical composition of pesticides.

8.5. Pesticides, between food and agricultural production

In order to place the discussions in a broader context, as well as the reflections which are sometimes considered when talking about pesticides, the corpus highlights the emergence of certain questions, in a non-exhaustive way:

– How are public health and financial health objectives linked in the case of pesticides?

– What is the relationship between pesticides and the dynamics of agricultural production?

– In terms of public health, how is legislation evolving, including at the European level?

– How do the farmers' working conditions factor into these discussions?

These questions are on everyone's lips, each with several different preconceptions including online, where Internet users deal with them in different ways, often (but not exclusively) depending on their political views: for example, between the *Reporterre* Facebook page and that of *Valeurs Actuelles*, the content of comments varies quite a bit. The results extracted from the corpus support this hypothesis.

The visualizations and analyses enabled by Iramuteq should not obscure the fact that it is always and systematically necessary to return to the corpus; i.e. to textual materials, which highlight situations of expression without attributing the study to the possibilities offered by the digital tool. Of course, as already emphasized, computer processing of the corpus allows us to consider the degree of frequency of lexical occurrences, and thus to study them in context. In other words, the measurement of these occurrences must be understood as a moment in the study when the occurrences can constitute many indications and entry points, which then enable us to return to the texts, allowing us to understand their semantic nuances.

8.6. A variety of positions

If we take the most characteristic segments of the corpus (in other words, those that use a significant combination of high-frequency occurrences), based on the calculation capabilities offered by Iramuteq, we can extract the following example, which contains seven quotes:

– "Which helps reduce the use of plant protection products; the nasty pesticides, GMOs as they say, have been used in medicine for decades and they save lives! Are you sure you are not fighting the wrong battle and missing the facts?" (comment from the Greenpeace Facebook page, about an article on the use of glyphosate in Mexico).

– "The majority of today's agriculture is contaminated by dangerous chemical substances. Do you want to remove pesticides and other products that are harmful to public health? It is possible, just get a law enacted that stipulates this" (comment from *Le Monde Afrique* YouTube page, about a video on the use of pesticides around Kinshasa).

– "The ending with the apple sprayed with pesticides seems exaggerated, but I'm afraid it is quite true. It is sad, there are so many shortcuts used, organic farming uses very dangerous products like copper" (comment from the *Amis des Lobbies* YouTube page, about a video on pesticide lobbying).

– "I am talking about agriculture, plant protection products are not only used by farmers, it is impressive how much plant protection products are used at home" (comment from *Arte*'s Facebook page, about a publication on the challenges of agriculture).

– "I mean, when you are pregnant, you do not use dangerous or toxic products: a herbicide, with or without glyphosate, is dangerous for anyone who handles it, and I am in no way clearing Monsanto and company" (comment from Konbini's YouTube page, about a video on the links between deformities and pesticides).

– "What I point out in their documentary is that they use the word *pesticide*, which can cause confusion with people, because in the general term, when we speak of pesticide, we think of industrial chemicals" (comment from the *Le Parisien* Facebook page, about an article on the presence of pesticides in raclette cheese).

– "Organic farming is a method of agricultural production that excludes the use of most synthetic chemicals: there are just as many, if not often more, pesticides in organic products than in nonorganic ones" (comment from the *Amis des Lobbies* YouTube page, about a video on pesticide lobbying).

The diversity of these positions speaks volumes, not just about the expressive attitudes of individuals in the digital comments but also about the representations surrounding pesticides, perceived either as a public health hazard requiring strong political intervention or as an element of technological progress, making it possible to feed the population, very often in a comparison with organic farming, which is represented in a negative way. This is particularly true of the first quotation, which also mixes pesticides and genetically modified organisms, combining the two in a positive light of technological and industrial innovation. In this type of case, some users use pesticide controversies to divert attention to the subject of comparing two agricultural models. In this situation of expression, the reader is forced to take a stance in favor of "reasonable" agriculture (in other words, with chemical pesticides) and "deceptive" agriculture (a priori without chemical pesticides). Discourse and counter-discourse clash around this theme.

More generally, the corpus reveals a number of discursive situations to questions and controversies linked to the presence and use of pesticides, particularly in agriculture, and therefore inevitably in consumer products (not to mention soil and air pollution, linked to the practice of spraying). A systemic analysis of the discourse, based in particular on identifying argumentative patterns, enables us to isolate six types of comments (and therefore of reactions) related to the theme of pesticides:

– Accepting pesticides through changing target:

- "We would eat a good raclette even if it had pesticides, they piss us off these ecologists and vegans. They should eat their herbs and processed products and leave us in peace" (comment from the *Le Parisien* Facebook page, on the presence of pesticides in raclette cheese).

- "Just so you know, organic farming uses tons of pesticides sold by Bayer" (comment from Hugo Clément's Facebook page, about Christmas tree farming).

– The nuance:

- "Indeed, chemical fertilizers and pesticides are so deeply rooted in our agricultural model that it would be complicated to abruptly withdraw them" (comment from Hugo Clément's Facebook page, about the use of glyphosate).

– Opposition or ban:

- "Pesticides are destroying our land and killing people. We must stop immediately! We cannot wait any longer" (comment from Hugo Clément's Facebook page, about the use of glyphosate).

- "It is about time everyone took some responsibility! No one is forcing consumers to eat pesticides" (comment from Hugo Clément's Facebook page, about the use of glyphosate).

– Diversion or conspiracy:

- "So, the pesticide yes, but the vaccine no?" (comment from the *Le Parisien* Facebook page, about the presence of pesticides in raclette cheese).

- "After the government wants us to believe that it wants to save us from Covid and poisons us with pesticides… it is worth thinking about… isn't it?" (comment from Hugo Clément's Facebook page, about the use of glyphosate).

– Humor:

- "We ate pesticides for lunch" (comment from the *Le Parisien* Facebook page, about the presence of pesticides in raclette cheese).

– Insults:

- "Go and drown yourself in your vats of pesticides 😮 We do not need farmers to feed ourselves" (comment from Hugo Clément's Facebook page, about Christmas tree farming).

These different families of comments, beyond the in-depth conversations on technical issues, reveal the representations that circulate within conversations about pesticides. Even if the fourth type of comments, related to the Covid-19 crisis, may seem out of step with the others, the fact remains that the subject of pesticides is sufficiently significant to relate with other social issues, generating scientific, political and social interdiscursive connections. In such cases, even if the issues often appear mixed, they are nonetheless significant from the perspective of political and social treatment.

8.7. Main themes

More generally, based on the results of Iramuteq and the linguistic material of the corpus, we distinguish five themes that Internet users gravitate toward with regard to pesticides: 1) food and consumption; 2) interactions and investigation; 3) the science of pesticides; 4) environmental effects; and 5) living with pesticides. The following specifics are developed:

– Food and consumption: on Facebook in particular, Internet users debate the impact of pesticides on food (or not), and their effects on health. Controversy not only comes up over the use of other products on organic produce but also over the capacity to produce enough to feed the entire population (which is linked to the scope of innovation and progress, from the view of pesticide advocates).

– Interaction and investigation: on YouTube in particular, videos attempt to explain what pesticides are, prompting interaction (appreciation) with the pages that put the videos online, while simultaneously praising the investigative approach to the subject, which shows that citizens want and need to know more. Here, videos can cover a wide range of subjects (from pesticide production and use to health effects), and these types of content systematically generate appreciative reactions.

– The science of pesticides: traditionally, in comparison to the other publications in our corpus, Reddit hosts more technical discussions on how pesticides actually work, giving rise to exchanges on chemistry, the impact on plant growth and the environment with lively debates, but which can also take place on other platforms, especially when they are led by individuals who clearly defend the use of pesticides and today's intensive agriculture (taking a stand against organic farming).

– Environmental effects: the impact of pesticides on nature is discussed in a versatile way, with obvious reference to their effects on soils, animal species – living organisms in general – the quality of cultivated species and the environment, as well as agricultural yields. Therefore, Roundup and neonicotinoid pesticides are mentioned in a resolutely ecological stance, which is highlighted within the corpus.

– Living with pesticides: a particularly interesting element is the fact that several individuals speak of living next to fields and crops sprayed with pesticides by farmers, while organic farmers report pesticide attacks on their land. This social aspect is highlighted several times and shows both a real tension between two agricultural models and between two representations of what life in rural areas should be (notably, the opposition between an imaginary healthy life, without danger to health, and a life with pesticides as health-damaging farm inputs).

These specific themes relate discourse and counter-discourse in a conversational way that sets the pace for controversy surrounding pesticides. In particular, their usefulness in the development of today's agricultural model is demonstrated, while also highlighting the tensions between two distinct agricultural models, as well as positive representations around notions of innovation and scientific progress, for those who support the use of pesticides (where those who oppose them arouse representations linked to ecology, the "natural" ("authentic", without being chemically altered by humans) aspect of food, rural life and health).

8.8. Conclusion

The online handling of discussions around pesticides explains the post-digital aspect of our society (Cramer 2015), which theorizes the absence of boundaries and the overcoming of limits between "reality" and "virtual", or "online" and "offline"; moreover, social networks enable social issues to be understood in the Web 2.0 era (Herring 2013), from both an interactional and a co-creative perspective. In other words, individuals engage in discursive activity, interact about it, allowing these discourses to go beyond digital devices into social debates, while at the same time reflecting and fueling them.

On the contrary, and in this specific context, the discourses and counter-discourses on pesticides are mostly made from the perspective of health, food and neighborhood life, which shows that they directly involve the daily lives of citizens, and that this interest in investigation shows a desire to know more on this subject, and probably on others too (notably because Web 2.0 allows direct interaction with those who are investigating). This is also what our study shows: while interactions between Internet users are particularly important in comments under articles and videos, these same Internet users are also in demand and in an expressive position for interaction when compared to the person or page publishing the videos or articles, particularly in the case of documentaries that inform and provide keys to understanding the pesticide issue.

Within these interactions, the individuals who comment use a relatively diverse range of argumentative positions, depending on the discourses or counter-discourses embodied in the linguistic material they use. The semantic productions and pragmatic devices used by Internet users are thus particularly varied and reflect the complexity of the controversy. From a general point of view, this complexity is expressed through concern or doubt about pesticides, or even denial of the potential risks, in a stance that can appear to be ideological on both sides. In this configuration, there is very little room for nuance. We hypothesize that the affordances of digital devices invite clear positions to be taken, conveying ideas that are sufficiently comprehensible so that they too can invite others to comment, share or react (through *likes*). In this regard, it is necessary to link discourse analysis to a critical analysis of the media devices that restrict the production of these discourses (Dahlberg 2013), if these devices also help to create communities that may voice their differences in discursive terms, thus reinforcing networks (Lo Monaco and Lheureux 2007; Lo Monaco et al. 2007) which encourage the maintenance of social bubbles, even in a post-digital context in which boundaries can seem blurred, or even invisible.

Lastly, the complexity of this network of discourses and counter-discourses around pesticides also highlights the unique media treatment given to the different spheres of influence that operate around this issue: depending on how the media present Monsanto, food issues, other public health controversies or the organic farming aspect, the stance people take varies considerably (e.g. a change of target, an attack on an ecologist or vegan movements, without, however, addressing the danger posed by certain molecules in the composition of pesticides). Therefore, while Internet users' comments reflect the discourses and counter-discourses in circulation, they also help to shape them, to alter the ways they are perceived and to bring them into conflict by creating content which, rather than helping to understand the complexity of an issue such as pesticides, tends to encourage communities to be structured. Ultimately, these communities are more concerned with their position and reinforcing themselves around key themes, due to the strong interactional aspect of social networks which we have highlighted, rather than seeking to identify the issues that would enable us to resolve this issue, which affects several aspects of our daily lives. Whether it is a question of health, food or agriculture, pesticides are, above all – at least on social networks – a distorted reflection of the state of social relations and of how they are mentioned through discourses and counter-discourses, at the heart of the mechanisms that promote them.

8.9. References

Alexander, A. (2009). *Framing Discourse on the Environment: A Critical Discourse Approach*. Routledge, London.

Amossy, R. (2011). Des sciences du langage aux sciences sociales : l'argumentation dans le discours. *A Contrario*, 16(2), 10–25.

Andersen, C.U., Cox, G., Papadopoulos, G. (2014). Postdigital research – Editorial. *A Peer-Reviewed Journal About*, 3(1), 4–7.

Angenot, M. (1977). Présupposé, topos, idéologème. *Le lieu commun*, 13(1/2), 11–34.

Baker, P. (2006). *Using Corpora in Discourse Analysis*. Continuum, London.

Barbazan, M. (2011). 'Enonciation' ou 'représentation du monde' ? Le jeu dynamique de la construction du sens dans les échanges verbaux. *Cahiers de praxématique*, 56, 117–166.

Bendinelli, M. (2011). Anglais de spécialité et logométrie. L'exemple des débats présidentiels américains. *Asp*, 60, 103–123.

Benhabib, S. (2002). *The Claims of Culture: Equality and Diversity in the Global Era*. Princeton University Press, Princeton.

Biros, C. (2014). Les couleurs du discours environnemental. *Mots. Les langages du politique*, 105, 45–66.

Calabrese, L. (2014). Rectifier le discours d'information médiatique. Quelle légitimité pour le discours profane dans la presse d'information en ligne ? *Les carnets du CEDISCOR*, 12, 21–34.

Campion, B. (2019). Glyphosate : l'impossible débat ? *La revue nouvelle*, 5(5), 71–82.

Charaudeau, P. (2007). Analyse du discours et communication. L'un dans l'autre ou l'autre dans l'un ? *Semen*, 23. doi: 10.4000/semen.5081.

Collet, C. and Charreton, M. (2017). Evaluation des capacités locomotrices de l'abeille en laboratoire : une méthode qui permet d'identifier des effets sublétaux après exposition à des pyréthrinoïdes et des néonicotinoïdes. *Innovations agronomiques*, 53, 105–109.

Cramer, F. (2015). What is 'post-digital' ? In *Postdigital Aesthetics: Art, Computation and Design*, Berry, D. and Dieter, M. (eds). Palgrave MacMillan, London, 12–26.

Dahlberg, L. (2013). Discourse theory as critical media politics? Five questions. In *Discourse Theory and Critical Media Politics*, Dahlberg, L. and Phelan, S. (eds). Palgrave Macmillan, London, 41–63.

Fairclough, N. (1992). *Discourse and Social Change*. Polity Press, Cambridge.

Fracchiolla, B. (2019). Ecologie et environnement : des mots aux discours. Mises en perspective historiques et discursives. *Mots. Les langages du politique*, 119.

Frants, V.I., Shapiro, J., Taksa, I., Voiskunskii, V.G. (1999). Boolean search: Current state and perspectives. *Journal of the American Society for Information Science*, 50(1), 86–95.

Garric, N. and Longhi, J. (2013). Atteindre l'interdiscours par la circulation des discours et du sens. *Langage et société*, 144(2), 65–83.

Hart, C. (2013). Argumentation meets adapted cognition: Manipulation in media discourse on immigration. *Journal of Pragmatics*, 59(2), 200–209.

Herring, S. (2013). Discourse in Web 2.0 familiar, reconfigured, and emergent. In *Discourse 2.0: Language and New Media*, Tannen, D. and Trester, A.M. (eds). Georgetown University Press, Washington, 1–26.

Howarth, D. (2000). *Discourse*. Open University Press, Buckingham.

Hwong, Y.-L., Oliver, C., Van Kranendonk, M., Sammut, C., Seroussi, Y. (2017). What makes you tick? The psychology of social media engagement in space science communication. *Computers in Human Behavior*, 68, 480–492.

Jouzel, J.-N. (2019). *Pesticides : comment ignorer ce que l'on sait*. Presses de Sciences Po, Paris.

Kopytowska, M. (2015). Mediating identity, ideology and values in the public sphere: Towards a new model of (constructed) social reality. *Lodz Papers in Pragmatics*, 11(2), 133–156.

Ledouble, H. (2020). Term circulation and conceptual instability in the mediation of science: Binary framing of the notions of biological versus chemical pesticides. *Discourse & Communication*, 14, 466–488.

Lo Monaco, G. and Lheureux, F. (2007). Représentations sociales : théorie du noyau central et méthodes d'étude. *Revue électronique de psychologie sociale*, 1, 1–55.

Lo Monaco, G., Rateau, P., Guimelli, C. (2007). Nexus, représentations sociales et masquage des divergences intra et intergroupes. *Bulletin de psychologie*, 6(492), 581–592.

Maillat, D. (2013). Constraining context selection: On the pragmatic inevitability of manipulation. *Journal of Pragmatics*, 59(2), 190–199.

Marchand, P. (1998). *L'analyse du discours assistée par ordinateur*. Armand Colin, Paris.

Martinez, W. (2012). Au-delà de la cooccurrence binaire… Poly-cooccurrences et trames de cooccurrence. *Corpus*, 11, 191–216.

Moirand, S. (2007). *Les discours de la presse quotidienne : observer, analyser, comprendre*. PUF, Paris.

Née, E. and Veniard, M. (2012). Analyse du Discours à Entrée Lexicale (A.D.E.L.) : le renouveau par la sémantique ? *Langage et société*, 140(2), 15–28.

Paveau, M.-A. (2006). *Les prédiscours : sens, mémoire, cognition*. Presses Sorbonne Nouvelle, Paris.

Reinert, M. (1990). ALCESTE – une méthodologie d'analyse des données textuelles et une application : Aurélia de Gérard de Nerval. *Bulletin de méthodologie sociologique*, 26, 24–54.

Reyna, J., Hanham, J., Meier, P. (2018). The Internet explosion, digital media principles and implications to communicate effectively in the digital space. *E-Learning and Digital Media*, 15(1), 36–52.

Rose, E. (2012). Hyper attention and the rise of the antinarrative: Reconsidering the future of narrativity. *Narrative Works: Issues, Investigations & Interventions*, 2(2), 92–102.

Rouquette, S. (2016). Aux marges de l'espace public médiatique. L'espace des commentaires des articles de presse en ligne. *Politiques de communication*, 6(1), 81–111.

Stewart, M. and Arnold, C. (2018). Defining social listening: Recognizing an emerging dimension of listening. *International Journal of Listening*, 32(2), 85–100.

Tournier, M. (1985). Texte 'propagandiste' et cooccurrences. Hypothèses et méthodes pour l'étude de la sloganisation. *Mots. Les langages du politique*, 11, 155–187.

Wagener, A. (2018). Discours politiques et dispositifs numériques : vers une nouvelle tectonique de la communication. *Neuphilologische Mitteilungen*, 119(2), 309–326.

Wagener, A. (2019). *Discours et système : théorie systémique du discours et analyse des représentations*. Peter Lang, Brussels.

Wagener, A. (2020). Hypernarrativity, storytelling, and the relativity of truth: Digital semiotics of communication and interaction. *Postdigital Science and Education*, 2(1), 147–169.

List of Authors

François ALLARD-HUVER
CHUS
Université Catholique de l'Ouest
Angers
France

Estera BADAU
CIMEOS
Université de Bourgogne
Dijon
France

Carole BARTHÉLÉMY
Laboratoire Population
Environnement Développement
Aix-Marseille Université
France

José Ramón BERTOMEU SÁNCHEZ
IILP
University of Valencia
Spain

Antoine BLANCHARD
Independent researcher
Bordeaux

Nataly BOTERO
CARISM
Université Paris-Panthéon-Assas
France

Eve BUREAU-POINT
Centre Norbert-Elias, CNRS
Aix-Marseille Université
France

Louis GALEY
LAPPS
Université Paris Nanterre
France

Alain GARRIGOU
EPICENE–BPH
INSERM
Université de Bordeaux
France

Fabienne GOUTILLE
EPICENE–BPN
Université de Bordeaux
France

Hélène LEDOUBLE
Babel
Université de Toulon
France

Annie MARTIN
SAGE
Université de Strasbourg
France

Clémence RAMBAUD
EPICENE
Université de Bordeaux
France

Jan SMOLINSKI
SAGE
Université de Strasbourg
France

Laurence THERY
Anact
Amiens
France

Albin WAGENER
Icam – Chaire Sens et Travail
and
PLIDAM
and
Université Catholique de Lille
and
PREFICS
France

Index

Other titles from

iSTE

in

Science, Society and New Technologies

2024

BARTHES Angela, CIBIEN Catherine, ROMAGNY Bruno
Biosphere Reserves and Sustainable Development Goals 1: Scientific and Practical Educational Issues in the Mediterranean
(Territory Development Set – Volume 3)
Biosphere Reserves and Sustainable Development Goals 2: Issues, Tensions, Processes and Governance in the Mediterranean
(Territory Development Set – Volume 4)

CATELLANI Andrea, LITS Grégoire
Transitions in Tension: Controversies and Tensions Around Ecological Transitions
(Communication, Environment, Science and Society Set – Volume 3)

DAVALLON Jean
Heritage Traces in the Making: A Communicational Analysis of Modes of Heritagization
(Traces Set – Volume 6)

DEJEAN Maxime, L'HOSTIS Marine, LI Meng
Chinese Outbound Tourism: From Source Markets to Destinations
(Tourism and Mobility Systems Set – Volume 8)

GAY Jean-Christophe
Tourismophobia: From "Mass Tourism" to "Overtourism"
(Tourism and Mobility Systems Set – Volume 9)

JULIA Guilhem, FAUCHON Anne, KANAWATI Rushed
AI, Healthcare and Law

KOHLMANN Émilie
Linking with Nature in the Digital Age
(Communication, Environment, Science and Society Set – Volume 1)

LEDOUBLE Hélène
Popularizing Science: The Complex Terminological Interactions between Scientific and Press Discourses within the Field of Agroecology
(Communication, Environment, Science and Society Set – Volume 2)

LOUART Pierre, PIRIOU Jérôme, VIOLIER Philippe
Tourist Destinations According to Stakeholder Strategies: From Clusters to Local Tourist Systems
(Tourism and Mobility Systems Set – Volume 7)

2023

APCHAIN Thomas
Favela Tours: Building Otherness in the Favelas of Rio de Janeiro
(Tourism and Mobility Systems Set – Volume 6)

CARDON Alain, EL HAMI Abdelkhalak
Fundamental Generation Systems: Computer Science and Artificial Consciousness, the Informational Field of Generation of the Universe, the Sixth Sense of Living Beings
(Digital Sciences Set – Volume 4)

CURULLI Irene G., IKIZ KAYA Deniz, KHAEFI Arghavan
Heritage Education for Climate Action
(Research in Architectural Education Set – Volume 2)

ELAMÉ Esoh
The Sustainable City in Africa Facing the Challenge of Liquid Sanitation
(Territory Development Set – Volume 2)

JURCZENKO Emmanuel
Climate Investing: New Strategies and Implementation Challenges

LYUBAREVA Inna, WALDECK Roger
Diversity of Methodological Approaches in Social Sciences: Example of the Analysis of Media and Online Information
(Modeling Methodologies in Social Sciences Set – Volume 3)

PARET Dominique, CRÉGO Pierre, SOLÈRE Pauline
Smart Patches: Biosensors, Graphene and Intra-Body Communications

VENTRE Daniel, GUILLOT Philippe
Electronic Communication Interception Technologies and Issues of Power

VENTRE Daniel, LOISEAU Hugo
Cybercrime during the SARS-CoV-2 Pandemic (2019-2022): Evolutions, Adaptations, Consequences
(Cybersecurity Set – Volume 3)

2022

AIT HADDOU Hassan, TOUBANOS Dimitri, VILLIEN Philippe
Ecological Transition in Education and Research

CARDON Alain
Information Organization of The Universe and Living Things: Generation of Space, Quantum and Molecular Elements, Coactive Generation of Living Organisms and Multiagent Model
(Digital Sciences Set – Volume 3)

CAULI Marie, FAVIER Laurence, JEANNAS Jean-Yves
Digital Dictionary

DAVERNE-BAILLY Carole, WITTORSKI Richard
Research Methodology in Education and Training: Postures, Practices and Forms
(Education Set – Volume 12)

ELAMÉ Esoh
Sustainable Intercultural Urbanism at the Service of the African City of Tomorrow
(Territory Development Set – Volume 1)

FLEURET Sébastien
A Back and Forth Between Tourism and Health: From Medical Tourism to Global Health
(Tourism and Mobility Systems Set – Volume 5)

KAMPELIS Nikos, KOLOKOTSA Denia
Smart Zero-energy Buildings and Communities for Smart Grids
(Engineering, Energy and Architecture Set – Volume 9)

2021

BARDIOT Clarisse
Performing Arts and Digital Humanities: From Traces to Data
(Traces Set – Volume 5)

BENSRHAIR Abdelaziz, BAPIN Thierry
From AI to Autonomous and Connected Vehicles: Advanced Driver-Assistance Systems (ADAS)
(Digital Sciences Set – Volume 2)

BÉRANGER Jérôme
Societal Responsibility of Artificial Intelligence: Towards an Ethical and Eco-responsible AI
(Technological Prospects and Social Applications Set – Volume 4)

CORDELIER Benoit, GALIBERT Oliver
Digital Health Communications
(Technological Prospective and Social Applications Set – Volume 5)

DOUAY Nicolas, MINJA Michael
Urban Planning for Transitions

GALINON-MÉLÉNEC Béatrice
The Trace Odyssey 1: A Journey Beyond Appearances
(Traces Set – Volume 4)

HENRY Antoine
Platform and Collective Intelligence: Digital Ecosystem of Organizations

KOLOKOTSA Denia, KAMPELIS Nikos
Smart Buildings, Smart Communities and Demand Response
(Engineering, Energy and Architecture Set – Volume 8)

LE LAY Stéphane, SAVIGNAC Emmanuelle, LÉNEL Pierre, FRANCES Jean
The Gamification of Society
(Research, Innovative Theories and Methods in SSH Set – Volume 2)

RADI Bouchaïb, EL HAMI Abdelkhalak
Optimizations and Programming: Linear, Non-linear, Dynamic, Stochastic and Applications with Matlab
(Digital Sciences Set – Volume 1)

2020

ALAKTIF Jamila, CALLENS Stéphane
Migration and Climate Change: From the Emergence of Human Cultures to Contemporary Management in Organizations

BARNOUIN Jacques
The World's Construction Mechanism: Trajectories, Imbalances and the Future of Societies
(Interdisciplinarity Between Biological Sciences and Social Sciences Set – Volume 4)

ÇAĞLAR Nur, CURULLI Irene G., SIPAHIOĞLU Işıl Ruhi, MAVROMATIDIS Lazaros E.
Thresholds in Architectural Education
(Engineering, Energy and Architecture Set – Volume 7)

DUBOIS Michel J.F.
Humans in the Making: In the Beginning was Technique
(Social Interdisciplinarity Set – Volume 4)

ETCHEVERRIA Olivier
The Restaurant, A Geographical Approach: From Invention to Gourmet Tourist Destinations
(Tourism and Mobility Systems Set – Volume 3)

GREFE Gwenaëlle, PEYRAT-GUILLARD Dominique
Shapes of Tourism Employment: HRM in the Worlds of Hotels and Air Transport
(Tourism and Mobility Systems Set – Volume 4)

JEANNERET Yves
The Trace Factory
(Traces Set – Volume 3)

KATSAFADOS Petros, MAVROMATIDIS Elias, SPYROU Christos
Numerical Weather Prediction and Data Assimilation
(Engineering, Energy and Architecture Set – Volume 6)

MARTI Caroline
Cultural Mediations of Brands: Unadvertization and Quest for Authority
(Communication Approaches to Commercial Mediation Set – Volume 1)

MAVROMATIDIS Lazaros
Climatic Heterotopias as Spaces of Inclusion: Sew Up the Urban Fabric
(Research in Architectural Education Set – Volume 1)

MOURATIDOU Eleni
Re-presentation Policies of the Fashion Industry: Discourse, Apparatus and Power
(Communication Approaches to Commercial Mediation Set – Volume 2)

SCHMITT Daniel, THÉBAULT Marine, BURCZYKOWSKI Ludovic
Image Beyond the Screen: Projection Mapping

VIOLIER Philippe, with the collaboration of TAUNAY Benjamin
The Tourist Places of the World
(Tourism and Mobility Systems Set – Volume 2)

2019

BRIANÇON Muriel
The Meaning of Otherness in Education: Stakes, Forms, Process, Thoughts and Transfers
(Education Set – Volume 3)

DESCHAMPS Jacqueline
Mediation: A Concept for Information and Communication Sciences
(Concepts to Conceive 21st Century Society Set – Volume 1)

DOUSSET Laurent, PARK Sejin, GUILLE-ESCURET Georges
Kinship, Ecology and History: Renewal of Conjectures
(Interdisciplinarity Between Biological Sciences and Social Sciences Set – Volume 3)

DUPONT Olivier
Power: A Concept for Information and Communication Sciences
(Concepts to Conceive 21st Century Society Set – Volume 2)

FERRARATO Coline
Prospective Philosophy of Software: A Simondonian Study
(Technological Prospects and Social Applications Set – Volume 3)

GUAAYBESS Tourya
The Media in Arab Countries: From Development Theories to Cooperation Policies

HAGÈGE Hélène
Education for Responsibility
(Education Set – Volume 4)

LARDELLIER Pascal
The Ritual Institution of Society
(Traces Set – Volume 2)

LARROCHE Valérie
The Dispositif: A Concept for Information and Communication Sciences
(Concepts to Conceive 21st Century Society Set – Volume 3)

LATERRASSE Jean
Transport and Town Planning: The City in Search of Sustainable Development

LELEU-MERVIEL Sylvie, SCHMITT Daniel, USEILLE Philippe
From UXD to LivXD: Living eXperience Design

LENOIR Virgil Cristian
Ethically Structured Processes
(Innovation and Responsibility Set – Volume 4)

LOPEZ Fanny, PELLEGRINO Margot, COUTARD Olivier
Local Energy Autonomy: Spaces, Scales, Politics
(Urban Engineering Set – Volume 1)

METZGER Jean-Paul
Discourse: A Concept for Information and Communication Sciences
(Concepts to Conceive 21st Century Society Set – Volume 4)

MICHA Irini, VAIOU Dina
Alternative Takes to the City
(Engineering, Energy and Architecture Set – Volume 5)

PÉLISSIER Chrysta
Learner Support in Online Learning Environments

PIETTE Albert
Theoretical Anthropology or How to Observe a Human Being
(Research, Innovative Theories and Methods in SSH Set – Volume 1)

PIRIOU Jérôme
The Tourist Region: A Co-Construction of Tourism Stakeholders
(Tourism and Mobility Systems Set – Volume 1)

PUMAIN Denise
Geographical Modeling: Cities and Territories
(Modeling Methodologies in Social Sciences Set – Volume 2)

WALDECK Roger
Methods and Interdisciplinarity
(Modeling Methodologies in Social Sciences Set – Volume 1)

2018

BARTHES Angela, CHAMPOLLION Pierre, ALPE Yves
Evolutions of the Complex Relationship Between Education and Territories
(Education Set – Volume 1)

BÉRANGER Jérôme
The Algorithmic Code of Ethics: Ethics at the Bedside of the Digital Revolution
(Technological Prospects and Social Applications Set – Volume 2)

DUGUÉ Bernard
Time, Emergences and Communications
(Engineering, Energy and Architecture Set – Volume 4)

GEORGANTOPOULOU Christina G., GEORGANTOPOULOS George A.
Fluid Mechanics in Channel, Pipe and Aerodynamic Design Geometries 1
(Engineering, Energy and Architecture Set – Volume 2)
Fluid Mechanics in Channel, Pipe and Aerodynamic Design Geometries 2
(Engineering, Energy and Architecture Set – Volume 3)

GUILLE-ESCURET Georges
Social Structures and Natural Systems: Is a Scientific Assemblage Workable?
(Social Interdisciplinarity Set – Volume 2)

LARINI Michel, BARTHES Angela
Quantitative and Statistical Data in Education: From Data Collection to Data Processing
(Education Set – Volume 2)

LELEU-MERVIEL Sylvie
Informational Tracking
(Traces Set – Volume 1)

SALGUES Bruno
Society 5.0: Industry of the Future, Technologies, Methods and Tools
(Technological Prospects and Social Applications Set – Volume 1)

TRESTINI Marc
Modeling of Next Generation Digital Learning Environments: Complex Systems Theory

2017

ANICHINI Giulia, CARRARO Flavia, GESLIN Philippe, GUILLE-ESCURET Georges
Technicity vs Scientificity: Complementarities and Rivalries (Interdisciplinarity Between Biological Sciences and Social Sciences Set – Volume 2)

DUGUÉ Bernard
Information and the World Stage: From Philosophy to Science, the World of Forms and Communications (Engineering, Energy and Architecture Set – Volume 1)

GESLIN Philippe
Inside Anthropotechnology: User and Culture Centered Experience (Social Interdisciplinarity Set – Volume 1)

GORIA Stéphane
Methods and Tools for Creative Competitive Intelligence

KEMBELLEC Gérald, BROUDOUX Evelyne
Reading and Writing Knowledge in Scientific Communities: Digital Humanities and Knowledge Construction

MAESSCHALCK Marc
Reflexive Governance for Research and Innovative Knowledge (Responsible Research and Innovation Set - Volume 6)

PARK Sejin, GUILLE-ESCURET Georges
Sociobiology vs Socioecology: Consequences of an Unraveling Debate (Interdisciplinarity Between Biological Sciences and Social Sciences Set – Volume 1)

PELLÉ Sophie
Business, Innovation and Responsibility (Responsible Research and Innovation Set – Volume 7)

2016

ANDRÉ Michel, SAMARAS Zissis
Energy and Environment
(Research for Innovative Transports Set – Volume 1)

BLANQUART Corinne, CLAUSEN Uwe, JACOB Bernard
Towards Innovative Freight and Logistics
(Research for Innovative Transports Set – Volume 2)

COHEN Simon, YANNIS George
Traffic Management
(Research for Innovative Transports Set – Volume 3)

EL FALLAH SEGHROUCHNI Amal, ISHIKAWA Fuyuki, HÉRAULT Laurent, TOKUDA Hideyuki
Enablers for Smart Cities

GIANNI Robert
Responsibility and Freedom: The Ethical Realm of RRI
(Responsible Research and Innovation Set – Volume 2)

GRUNWALD Armin
The Hermeneutic Side of Responsible Research and Innovation
(Responsible Research and Innovation Set – Volume 5)

LENOIR Virgil Cristian
Ethical Efficiency: Responsibility and Contingency
(Responsible Research and Innovation Set – Volume 1)

PELLÉ Sophie, REBER Bernard
From Ethical Review to Responsible Research and Innovation
(Responsible Research and Innovation Set – Volume 3)

REBER Bernard
Precautionary Principle, Pluralism and Deliberation: Science and Ethics
(Responsible Research and Innovation Set – Volume 4)

TORRENTI Jean-Michel, LA TORRE Francesca
Materials and Infrastructures 1
(Research for Innovative Transports Set – Volume 5A
Materials and Infrastructures 2
(Research for Innovative Transports Set – Volume 5B)

VENTRE Daniel
Information Warfare – 2nd edition

YANNIS George, COHEN Simon
Traffic Safety
(Research for Innovative Transports Set – Volume 4)

2015

BRONNER Gérald
Belief and Misbelief Asymmetry on the Internet

2009

VENTRE Daniel
Information Warfare

Printed and bound by CPI Group (UK) Ltd, Croydon, CR0 4YY
13/09/2026
14961048-0001